WAVEFRONT
A TEXT AND ATLAS

WAVEFRONT
A TEXT AND ATLAS

Editor

Roberto Pinelli MD
Scientific Director
Istituto Laser Microchirurgia Oculare
Brescia, Italy

Foreword

Tangwa Martin Neville

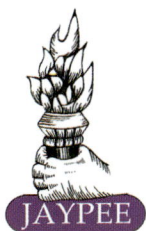

JAYPEE

JAYPEE BROTHERS MEDICAL PUBLISHERS (P) LTD

New Delhi • London • Philadelphia • Panama

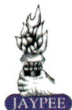

Jaypee Brothers Medical Publishers (P) Ltd.

Headquarters

Jaypee Brothers Medical Publishers (P) Ltd.
4838/24, Ansari Road, Daryaganj
New Delhi 110 002, India
Phone: +91-11-43574357
Fax: +91-11-43574314
Email: jaypee@jaypeebrothers.com

Overseas Offices

J.P. Medical Ltd.
83, Victoria Street, London
SW1H 0HW (UK)
Phone: +44-2031708910
Fax: +02-03-0086180
Email: info@jpmedpub.com

Jaypee-Highlights Medical Publishers Inc.
City of Knowledge, Bld. 237, Clayton
Panama City, Panama
Phone: +1 507-301-0496
Fax: +1 507-301-0499
Email: cservice@jphmedical.com

Jaypee Medical Inc.
The Bourse
111, South Independence Mall East
Suite 835, Philadelphia, PA 19106, USA
Phone: +1 267-519-9789
Email: jpmed.us@gmail.com

Jaypee Brothers Medical Publishers (P) Ltd.
17/1-B, Babar Road, Block-B, Shaymali
Mohammadpur, Dhaka-1207
Bangladesh
Mobile: +08801912003485
Email: jaypeedhaka@gmail.com

Jaypee Brothers Medical Publishers (P) Ltd.
Bhotahity, Kathmandu, Nepal
Phone: +977-9741283608
Email: kathmandu@jaypeebrothers.com

Website: www.jaypeebrothers.com
Website: www.jaypeedigital.com

Inquiries for bulk sales may be solicited at: jaypee@jaypeebrothers.com

Wavefront: A Text and Atlas

First Edition: **2014**

ISBN 978-93-5152-247-8

Printed at Ajanta Offset & Packagings Ltd., New Delhi

Dedicated to

All my colleagues

Contributors

Alfredo Vega Estrada MD
Ophthalmologist (Cornea and Refractive Surgery)
Division of Ophthalmology
Universidad Miguel Hernández
VISSUM Corporación Oftalmológica
Alicante, Spain

David S Chu MD
Assistant Professor
Department of Ophthalmology
University of Medicine and Dentistry of New Jersey (UMDNJ)
New Jersey Medical School
New Jersey
Ocular Disease Specialist
The Cornea and Laser Eye Institute—Hersh Vision Group
Teaneck, New Jersey, USA

Elena Scaffidi MA
Clinical Psychologist
Vision Psychology Service
Istituto Laser Microchirurgia Oculare
Brescia, Italy

Jesús Andrés Rosas Apráez MD
Professor
Refractive Surgery Unit
University Sanitas of Bogotá, Colombia

José Luis Güell MD
Professor
Department of Cornea and Refractive Surgery
Istituto de Microchirurgia Ocular
Barcelona, Spain

Jorge L Alio MD PhD
Founder of VISSUM Corporation
Professor and
Chairman of Ophthalmology
VISSUM Corporación Oftalmológica
Alicante, Spain

Juan Pablo Castañeda Borrero MD
Ophthalmic Surgeon
Clinical Colsanitas SA
Bogotá, Colombia

Luis Antonio Ruiz MD
Scientific Director
Centro Oftalmológico Colombiano
Bogotá, Colombia

Pablo Peña-García MD
Researcher
VISSUM Corporación Oftalmológica
Division of Ophthalmology
Universidad Miguel Hernández
Alicante, Spain

Peter S Hersh MD
Professor
Department of Clinical Ophthalmology
Director
Cornea and Refractive Surgery Division
New Jersey Medical School
The Cornea and Laser Eye Institute—Hersh Vision Group
Teaneck, New Jersey, USA

Roberto Pinelli MD
Scientific Director
Istituto Laser Microchirurgia Oculare
Brescia, Italy

Tangwa Martin Neville MD
Istituto Laser Microchirurgia Oculare
Brescia, Italy

Vance Thompson MD
Scientific Director
Refractive Surgery
Vance Thompson Vision
Sioux Falls, South Dakota, USA

Yazan A Zahran MD
Ophthalmologist and Refractive Surgeon
Dr Yazan Zahran Eye Clinic
Amman, Jordan

Yinfei Xu BS
The Cornea and Laser Vision Institute—Hersh Group
Teaneck, New Jersey, USA

Foreword

Wavefront: A Text and Atlas will give a personal light to the readers. Personal because it is showing personal experiences of refractive surgeons, clinical activity, and also, because it is showing a "panorama" or wavefront and aberrations "planet" without preconcepts, but based on elementary opinions, descriptions and cases.

To the reader the final judge, hopefully uncontaminated.

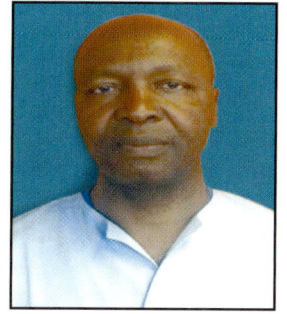

Tangwa Martin Neville MD
Istituto Laser Microchirurgia Oculare
Brescia, Italy

Preface

In our daily activity, the ophthalmologists as well as the optometrists have dealt with refractive errors—myopia, hyperopia, presbyopia, and various forms and combinations of astigmatisms. In terms of eye aberrations, they are part of the lower-order aberrations precisely of the second-order. Lower eye aberrations include piston tilt/prisms which are zero- and first-order, and together with the second-order are estimated to form 80/85% of all eye aberrations.

The second leg of this topic—the higher-order aberrations, have come into frequent use, and with the advent of and consolidation of refractive surgery, together with the commercialization of aberrometers. Further knowledge and insight into these aberrations has been attained.

However, aberrations are newcomer in our language and practice. The effort herein, which is quite elementary seeks to deal with and offer a handy consultation atlas, simple to read and easier to consult in our offices. While lower-order aberrations are manageable with spectacle glasses, contact lenses and refractive surgery. Higher-order aberrations though quite known and understood still have treatment far from offhand.

In the atlas, the readers will find a fluent descriptive part, some clinical examples and cases. At the end of all, a few graphical elaborations and clinical pictures retrieved from present and updated literature. The topic is in full debate and evolution. My desire was that simple—provide a manual and I hope that I have met the task.

Roberto Pinelli

Acknowledgment

Special thank to the entire team of Istituto Laser Microchirurgia Oculare, Brescia, Italy.

Contents

SECTION 1

The Project of Vision: Hypothesis for a Functional Structure

CHAPTER 1

Roberto Pinelli

A New Winning Philosophy

THE VISION INSTITUTE

Why do we describe ourselves as a 'vision institute' and not a 'refractive surgery center' or a general 'ophthalmology institute'.?

We refer to our center [the Istituto Laser Microchirurgia Oculare **(Fig. 1)**] as a 'vision institute': Refractive surgery represents its core business, but there are many other professionals involved who make their contribution to offer an excellent service from multidisciplinary perspectives in the vision field.

A vision institute is a health center entirely devoted to vision in all its aspects. All types of visual defect are treated by means of refractive surgery, employing a wide range of technology and a multidisciplinary medical and nonmedical team.

In addition, ophthalmological diseases are treated in accordance with the latest protocols. In this way, the ophthalmic patient is followed in each phase of his/her life, and can take the institute as a point of reference for ophthalmic health throughout life. Let us consider for example, a patient, 35-year-old, with –15D sph., –2D cyl. in both eyes.

His myopia can be resolved by implanting a phakic IOL, and the astigmatism can be subsequently dealt with by means of LASIK or ASA.

When he turns 60, he might develop a cataract: The phakic IOL can be removed at this point and substituted with an artificial lens through phacoemulsification. Presbyopia could be solved by the use of an accommodative IOL, or through corneal surgery (CK or P-curve) subsequent to lens implantation. If the patient presents any kind of problem with the health of his

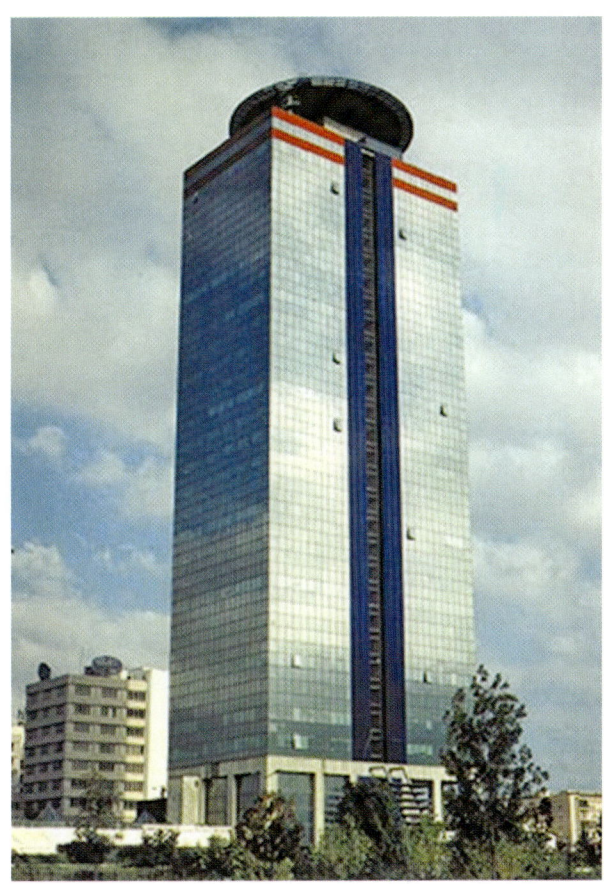

Fig. 1: Crystal palace, seat of the Istituto Laser Microchirurgia Oculare

eyes (retina, glaucoma, etc.), the vision institute offers him a state-of-the-art center at the forefront of research where he can be confident of receiving treatment from specialists who are continually updating their expertise.

Furthermore, the patient will be followed each step of the way by the psychologist who will monitor his/her emotional situation throughout, and will provide help in facing up to the changes that refractive surgery or a medical therapy may provoke not only without, but also within.

Thus, it is that vision in all its multifaceted meanings is to be considered the true core business of the institute, above and beyond 'mere' refractive surgery or ophthalmology.

STRUCTURE OF THE NEW VISION INSTITUTE

The Medical Staff

The medical staff within a vision institute comprises a number of professionals with different roles. Duties should be specifically allocated among each member of the medical staff in order that the different aspects of ophthalmology are covered.

The main aim of the assistants in ophthalmology is to clarify all the possible doubts that can arise for patients concerning their visual situation, analyzing it through the most innovative technologies. Furthermore, we believe that it is of primary importance to establish a relationship based on reliance with the patient, to make him feel at ease in each moment of his/her transit through the institute.

In conclusion, professionalism should always be accompanied by strong interpersonal skills, and for this reason we firmly believe nonmedical staff members should be fully trained in this area, stimulating the sense of belonging to a team united in the same purpose.

The Front Desk Staff

The first impression that patients have of the Institute is of paramount importance, since it initiates a complex series of judgments that will ideally remain positive in nature.

As soon as the patient enters the Institute he evaluates the setting, the courtesy of the staff, and their willingness to help. He also immediately realizes who it is that he can refer to, as the Front Desk (FD) and Patient Care (PC) staff wear a uniform providing a constant and unmistakable point of reference for the patient.

It may sound trivial but the uniform is an essential aspect of those staff members who are the first to come into direct contact with the patient (such as Front Desk and Patient Care staff).

The FD staff must help the patient to feel comfortable and at ease, always welcoming him with a smile and remembering

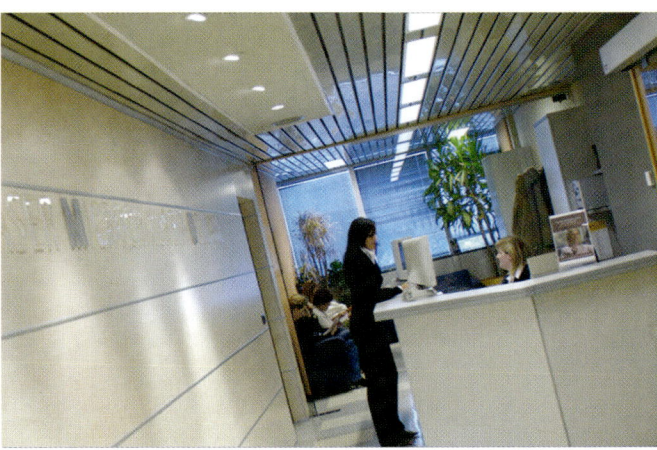

Fig. 2: The entrance of the institute

his name, offering a seat, a refreshing drink, and a choice of magazines **(Fig. 2)**.

On the occasion of the first examination at the Institute, for example, the patient is invited to answer some questions relating to his personal details with the help of the FD staff, whose duty is also to administer a questionnaire called the 'Questionnaire of symptoms' edited in collaboration with the Center for Functional Nutrition for Longevity.

The answers to the questionnaire allow the surgeon to gain a better understanding of the relationship between the visual condition of the patient and his general state of health and to provide more appropriate and customized instructions.

The FD staff is personally involved in the internal organization of the Institute: It has to schedule the agendas in an optimum way, striving to reduce waiting times during agenda management, daily consultations and surgery. Only this way we can obtain efficient team work that enables the best results to be achieved. This implies not only a good knowledge of the duties of the entire staff, but also the ability to anticipate the outcome of a visit, thereby planning its duration allocated in the agenda **(Fig. 3)**.

In general the day comprises general and preoperative examinations and check-ups (postoperative and others), scheduled in the agenda on the basis of the surgery conducted. Having set out the surgical calendar, the examination days are planned. Normally no examinations are scheduled during surgery day, in order that the whole staff (clinical and nonclinical), can devote themselves entirely to patient management. Even the day after surgery is organized so that the first part of the morning is reserved for those patients operated on the previous day.

Together with this procedure the FD staff has to be able to manage all the incoming calls: Some of these may involve altering the day or time of a fixed appointment, but most of them egard refractive surgery. The callers usually ask for information regarding: Time needed to fix a consultation,

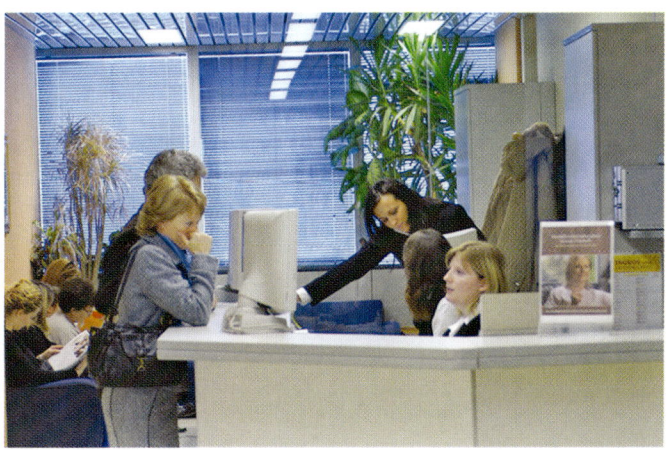

Fig. 3: The front desk with part of the staff

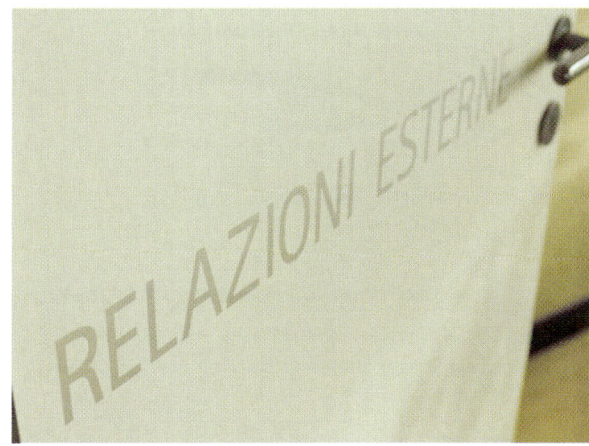

Fig. 4: The external relations department

What to do before the consultation, Cost of the visit and the time required for surgery if it is deemed appropriate.

It is obvious that the more we communicate with our callers the more open and honest will be the exchange of information. It is also important to underline that sometimes aspiring patients, are not necessarily good candidates for surgery—(see physical/clinical and motivational requirements assessed by the clinical and patient care staff).

The role of the FD staff is to be helpful, informative, relaxed, and cheerful where appropriate, but most of all they must possess a high degree of knowledge pertaining to of the specific subject and must transmit confidence: Only this way can one hope to gently persuade the patient to make an appointment for a consultation, without imposing any pressure so to do. FD staff must be able to discover, analyze and recognize patients emotional needs, state, fears, frustrations and be able to play an active role in the patient's exploration of options regarding refractive surgery. It may seem trivial, but not only does the choice of words used play an important role, but also the voice of the person speaking with the patient to establish communication. The importance of establishing true communication is highlighted in the preoperative phase during the interview with the PC staff.

The External Relations Department Between Information and Marketing

Marketing is one of the most important elements in a private company, and a portion of the budget needs to be constantly allocated to it.

A precise yearly plan regarding the use of the media to market the company services and products is fundamental for attracting customers and ensuring that the company reaches, and stays in, the public eye **(Fig. 4)**.

As far as a health company is concerned, marketing still remains an important expense, but some qualifications are necessary. First of all, it must be clear what we are talking about. We are not discussing marketing in a public health environment, such as a hospital or an emergency room for example. What leads people towards these places is necessity or urgency (pain, a sudden health problem, or the need for special services that only large public services can offer). This kind of health service cannot be compared to a private one, if we consider dimensions and core business.

The topic that we want to analyze in this chapter is marketing in a private health company that offers those services and practices that are not "urgent", that are not geared towards saving a patient's life. Of course, such health centers offer clinical practices that undoubtedly greatly improve a patient's quality of life, but they are not of primary importance for the continuation of life.

In this specific case, we aim to analyze the distinctive qualities of the external relations department of a vision institute, which offers different services and technologies to restore patients' vision. The external relations department must constantly maintain a fine balance between the need to promote services offered by the institute and the necessity to abide by the dictates of the law in this delicate matter. We will start by analyzing the Italian regulations for publicity in health.

The ethical code of conduct in professional practice of 1999 sums up the main legal concepts regarding publicity in health (which was the modification of a previous and more stringent law of 1992). It has been reported previously and gives us a clear idea of what the general trend of the law in Italy is: The medical doctor, in this case the refractive surgeon, shall not promote the public or private heath structure where he/she professionally operates, through the most common media (newspapers, magazines, television). Information in the health sector may not present any of the typical

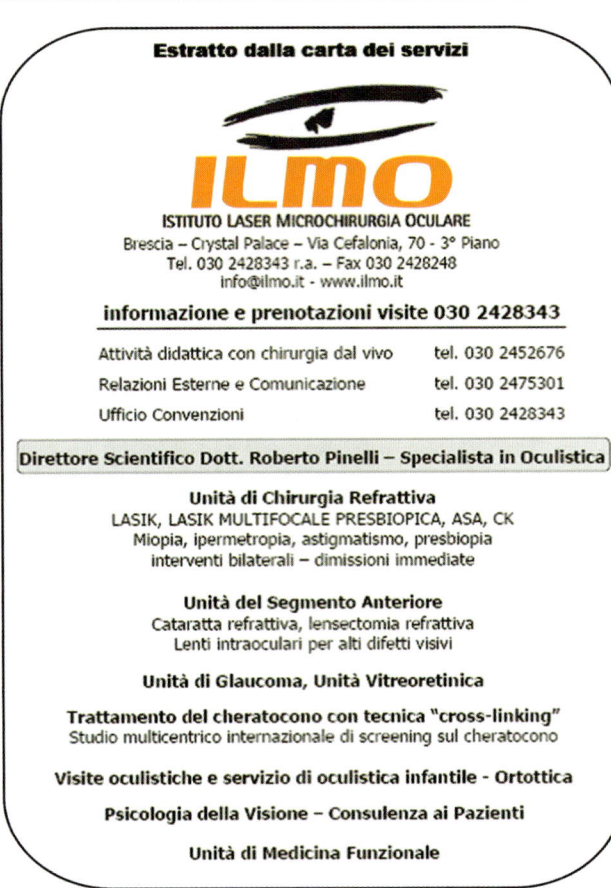

Fig. 5: Services information about the institute

features of commercial publicity **(Fig. 5)**. This is meant, of course, to guarantee a professional health system to all the citizens, avoiding the possibility that financial enterprise in health services could mitigate against quality in these same services. It is, of course, correct to regulate the marketing and the publicity in such a delicate area, considering that often people's lives depend on the quality of the services they get in hospitals or in private health companies.

As mentioned, the regulation in 1992 was even more stringent: The only kind of publicity allowed was the doorplate (with the name of the doctor and his/her academic titles) and informative articles only in sector publications. Furthermore, even the doorplate had to be approved by the Public Body and by the local Medical Board Association. In 1999 the law relaxed somewhat, additionally allowing doctors to publicise in any general magazine, including those publications that we usually find in bookshops. This made things easier for those companies that offered private health services, who could now use the media in a different and more profitable way.

Of course, the doctor is not completely free of bias and cannot say or write anything he likes in any newspaper or magazine, but now he has the possibility of publishing the

'Services Chart' of his private company without needing any permission to do so.

What is the most delicate issue in the external relations department of an innovative center such as a full service vision institute? The balance between scientific information (characterized by specificity of terms, mathematical and statistical analysis of data, and for this reason not really attractive to the public) and marketing (characterized on the contrary by a fresh and user-friendly language, colored pictures, easy concepts). This balance is sometimes very hard to find.

Concepts Vital to Every Marketing Initiative

- Professionalism
- High quality standards in all services offered
- Innovative technologies
- Particular and significant attention to the patient
- The patient is the center and always remains at the center
- Particular attention to national and international research
- Constant attention to contact with other similar centers in the world.

How can we Transmit all these Concepts Attractively and yet Still Abide by the Law?

Newspapers and Magazines

Articles appearing in local and national reviews are an excellent marketing tool that allow the surgeon and his institute to become known in his geographical and historical context. These articles must always be perfectly balanced in the sense that they must be easy to read but full of information. They must attract the reader's attention (through beautiful pictures, for example, that do not bring the mind to 'scary scenarios' often seen in the news), and keep the attention gained by providing useful and interesting information in a fresh way. Language is of primary and absolute importance: Nowadays readers are usually quite well informed, so they need to read texts written in an appropriate manner. On the other hand, the vocabulary used in the scientific reviews is often incomprehensible, and it would not fit a 'softer' contest such as a normal magazine **(Fig. 6)**.

Television

Television (TV) represents a powerful tool in marketing. There are many programs that concentrate on health, inviting nationally well-known professionals to discuss different problems or new therapies or technologies in various fields of medicine. Participation in these programs (usually greatly appreciated by the public) is usually part of a planned marketing strategy. In fact, it allows the institute to become very well known in a short time and over a large area. It is not possible (because of the previously discussed regulations) to display the name of the vision center on air. This is why,

LASIK in estate: perché no?

Non c'è stagione più o meno indicata per dire addio agli occhiali, quando tutti i parametri sono valutati da un chirurgo refrattivo esperto, in grado di determinare l'idoneità del paziente all'intervento di correzione di un difetto visivo - sia esso miopia, ipermetropia, astigmatismo o presbiopia - non ci sono particolari rischi, tanto meno quelli legati alla stagionalità, come il caldo, il vento, l'esposizione al sole, la vita all'aria aperta.

Se la visita diagnostica è eseguita correttamente, in base agli standard internazionali, e se non vengono rilevate controindicazioni, non c'è alcun bisogno di rimandare un intervento che invece può risultare molto utile proprio in vista di una vacanza estiva, magari all'insegna dello sport e dell'attività fisica. In una stagione in cui si cerca la libertà e lo svago, poter fare a meno degli occhiali è un vantaggio in più.

Senza dimenticare che, grazie alle tecniche prodotte dalla ricerca internazionale, oggi gli interventi di correzione dei difetti visivi si eseguono ambulatorialmente, non richiedono anestesia se non l'instillazione di alcune gocce di collirio, e permettono al paziente di riprendere le sue normali attività nel giro di un paio di giorni.

Al di là della stagione, ciò che è importante sapere è che la microchirurgia oculare italana è in alcuni centri ai migliori livelli tecnologici e clinici. Oggi è possibile trattare i difetti visivi con tecniche sicure ed efficaci, come la LASIK, proposta nei centri più all'avanguardia in versione bilaterale e simultanea, che consente al paziente di tornare a casa subito dopo l'intervento, indossando semplicemente un paio di occhiali da sole e consentendo di riprendere le attività consuete già dal giorno successivo all'intervento. L'operazione dura qualche minuto per occhio, è assolutamente indolore ed è sicura ed efficace.

L'arrivo dell'estate è uno stimolo verso l'indipendenza dagli occhiali. E' inoltre necessario dare un'informazione corretta a chi pensa di avvicinarsi a queste opportunità oferte dalla ricerca oculistica: la LASIK si può effettaure tutto l'anno. Dal punto di vista medico non vi è alcuna ragione per sconsigliare l'intervento in questo periodo dell'anno, se la tecnica è LASIK. Un paio di occhiali da sole che proteggono dai raggi del sole nei primi due o tre giorni dopo l'intervento sono l'unica accortezza richiesta a coloro che non vogliono rinunciare ad un'estate in tutta libertà.

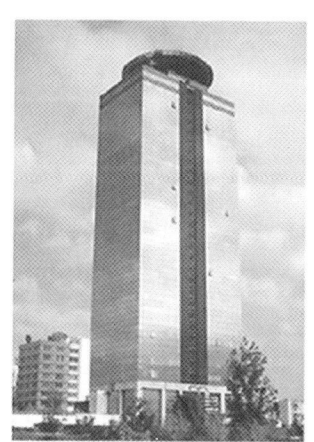

Dr. Roberto Pinelli
Direttore Scientifico
Istituto Laser Microchirurgia Oculare
Brescia

Fig. 6: An article about the institute published on a local newspaper

before investing in TV presence, it is important to have a solid and sound reputation and to occupy a prominent position on the web in order to be found easily.

Breaking News: The Patient Care Staff

The patients themselves have often painted an eloquent picture when describing the PC staff, whose principal characteristic is to offer the recognized value of a point of reference: A light at the end of the tunnel, a mountain guide, and a tutor.

The PC staff plays an essential role in an Institute devoted to the correction of visual defects. Its main aim is to provide patients with accurate and comprehensive information regarding surgery, often with a view to clearing up the confusion patients frequently have on the subject.

One of the main prerogatives of the Institute is to assist the patient affected by a visual problem or defect right through from the very first preoperative consultation to the last postoperative examination.

The PC staff aims to help the patient to understand his personal visual situation, his desires, his expectations and must also satisfy his requests and answer any questions he may have concerning surgery.

Assuming the patient's clinical suitability, could a patient nevertheless not reflect suitable 'psychological parameters' and have expectations which are incompatible with the results that refractive surgery could offer?

Confirmation of a patient's suitability for surgery is therefore made via an appropriate assessment of his/her motivation.

To evaluate the patient's motivation for the surgery the Patient Care staff must pay attention to his behavior during the consultation, assessing his expectations, doubts, desires and fears. To overcome fears of surgery for example, it is necessary to describe the procedure step by step to the patient, using appropriate terminology, method and tone of voice. It can also prove valuable to refer to the fact that some of the staff of the institute have also undergone eye surgery.

A MANAGEMENT HYPOTHESIS ON DAILY BRIEFING: CONTACTS BETWEEN MEDICAL AND NONMEDICAL STAFF (ANALYZING THE DAILY PATIENTS' AGENDA)

At the Istituto Laser Microchirurgia Oculare (ILMO) the day begins with a 'briefing' concerning the patients scheduled in the agenda **(Fig. 7)**. All staff members must attend, even those who do not normally come into direct contact with patients (for example the External Relations staff). The ILMO is of the firm conviction that anything concerning the work of the Institute involves everyone who works for it.

It is evident that people bringing different knowledge and different professions working in the same center can represent

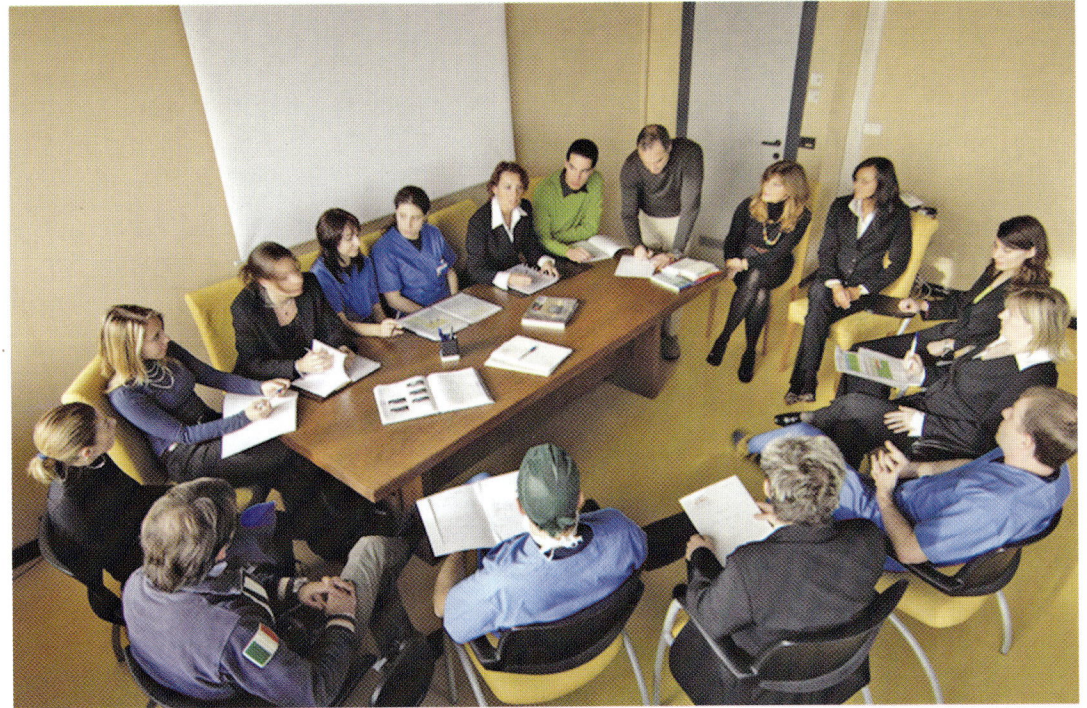

Fig. 7: The staff gathered in the meeting room

a wide gamut of important resources to meet patient's needs and can foster a co-operative working atmosphere.

This briefing allows the medical staff to enjoy a mutual exchange of ideas with the nonmedical staff and to strive to reach the optimal solution for each patient.

The FD (PC) staff knows much about the patient, not only through what is written in his case history (taken when he first came to the Institute) but also has an understanding of his true needs and whether he has particular fears, expectations or anxieties. Such elements can help the medical staff to satisfy such needs.

What makes the relationship between the medical and nonmedical staff relevant is that the FD staff is constantly evaluating and streamlining the management of timing during daily consultations with the consequence that patient waiting times are reduced **(Fig. 8)**.

The role of the FD staff is also to organize the movement of the patients within the Institute and thereby avoid bottleneck situations (often arising from high patient numbers) both in the waiting rooms and other areas. When patients arrive they are split into two waiting rooms and it is the task of the front desk staff to make note of those present and direct them to the appropriate examination rooms.

The logistics of patient management during surgery times changes rhythm fundamentally with respect to examination days. One of the two waiting rooms is dedicated to patients awaiting surgery and their accompanying persons; the other room is appropriately darkened to prevent any intense external light entering (an immediate postoperative requirement). This room is designed to receive the patient

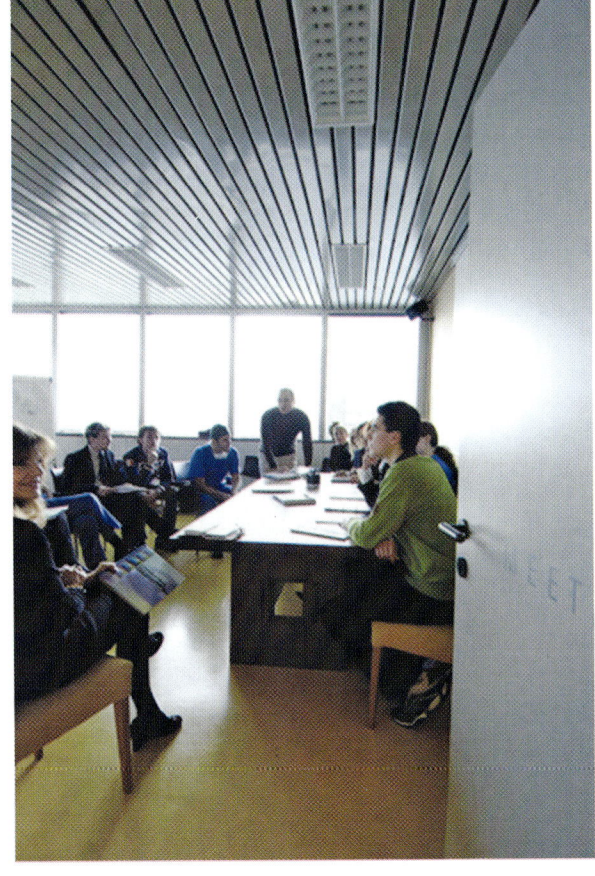

Fig. 8: Meetings take place to discuss the schedule of the day

after surgery, providing a reserved space which is calm and relaxing, where some time can be spent with those accompanying him, before they leave the Institute.

The medical staff has a great influence on the work of the FD because it can provide key education and training to impart specific knowledge which will prove especially useful when talking to the patient regarding treatment following the consultations or when managing patient needs in the immediate postoperative phase. During this particular phase, the patient needs to have a point of reference, somebody to talk to, and before speaking to the Patient Care staff (devoted to that very task) he can be sure that he is speaking to somebody who immediately understands him, and when and what kind of surgery he had. We could even talk of an 'art of listening' that characterizes the FD (and Patient Care staff). Not least because another vital aim is that of being able to recognize, from a description of symptoms on the phone, any potential complications (after surgery or after therapy) and so be in a position to provide appropriate medical advice.

CHAPTER 2

Roberto Pinelli

Highlights on Statistics and Clinical Research

EXTERNAL RELATIONS FOR SURGICAL AND CLINICAL NEWS

A continuous updating regarding both the latest technology and the results of research being conducted in other eye surgery centers in the world is surely one of the key factors contributing to the success of the vision institute. This is of primary importance for several reasons:

- Being at the forefront in terms of the latest ophthalmology treatments and state-of-the-art technology means that the institute provides a point of reference for all patients, who over time appreciate that the institute is indeed a full service vision center that employs the latest technology and treatment for any possible ophthalmic disease.
- To maintain contact with other eye centers worldwide, it is essential to be updated in the different research fields in ophthalmology. Moreover, it is very useful to compare one's own results with those of colleagues, in order to improve one's own services and ensure that the institute plays a significant role of at world level.
- Very often, in the scientific peer-reviewed journals in ophthalmology one can find interesting suggestions for the internal organization of the center from the marketing and administrative point of view (**Fig. 1**). Sometimes, expert administrators in the ophthalmic fields write or edit dedicated sections in such publications, offering well thought-out advice and describing existing exemplary models of vision centers. It is therefore important to study all the scientific publications carefully in order to draw inspiration from those innovations that could improve the internal organization of the institute, reinterpreting

such ideas in the light of the institute's own geographical, cultural and social setting.

As we have seen, it is of primary importance to pay particular attention to the scientific publications for many reasons. Here are some practical suggestions to make the most of them:

- First of all, the office manager of the institute should make sure that the institute subscribes to all the important, high-impact scientific journals. Some of these are strictly linked to scientific societies, and the subscription is automatic when the senior surgeon or a member of the staff joins the relevant society. Those journals whose subscriptions are not contingent upon society membership can be readily subscribed to online or by contacting the publisher directly. Many journals are also available online, and anybody can subscribe to a newsletter service that will automatically send to the requestor a regular summary of the main topics dealt with in each issue as and when it is published. In some cases it is possible to choose one's favorite topics and receive articles on those very topics on a regular basis by e-mail.
- Once the journals are in the institute they should be systematically reviewed by a designated staff member. A practical suggestion could be for example to copy the most interesting articles and distribute them to the appropriate department. In this way each member of the staff can be kept updated about the latest issues in ophthalmology with a particular emphasis on his or her own job. A knowledge of English is, of course, of primary importance, as all the international scientific journals are published in English.

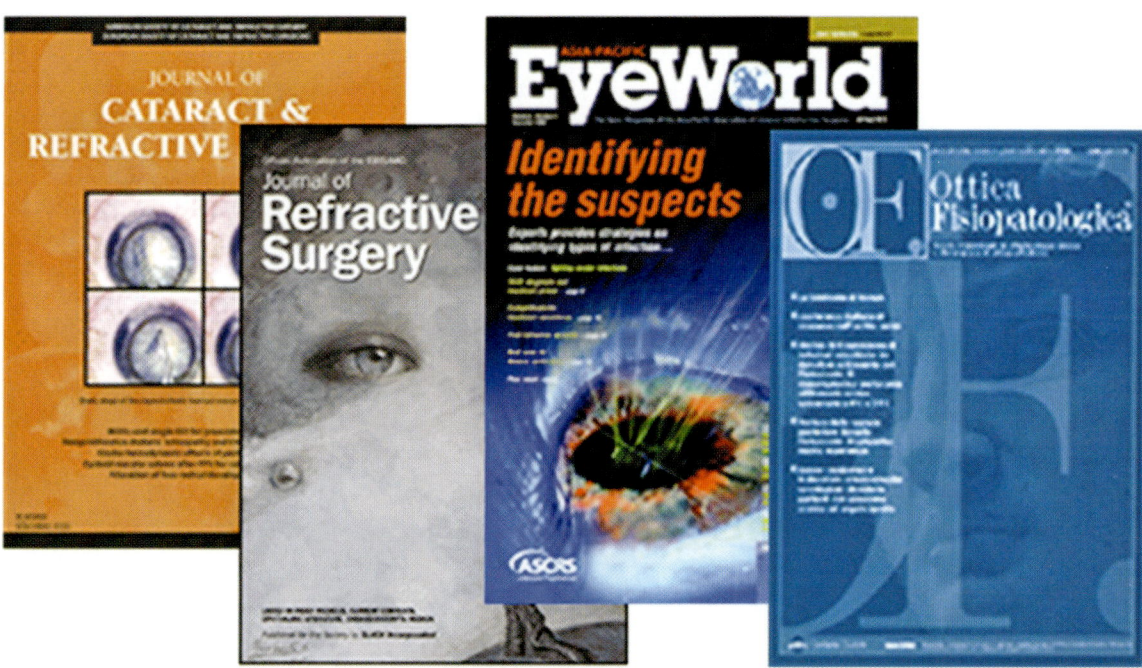

Fig. 1: Some of the most important journals about refractive surgery

- Furthermore, it is useful to devote a period in the weekly or monthly schedule of the institute (depending on the surgical and examination agendas) to a discussion of those articles, in a 'journal club'. Each member of the staff can periodically choose a topic, collect the most interesting articles and describe it to the colleagues from a critical point of view. It offers the whole team a chance to discuss and acquire knowledge about the colleague's department, and to gain a wider view of the topic as a result of studying international contributions to research in the sector.

So far, we have only discussed the scientific periodical publications in ophthalmology. Equal attention should obviously be paid to books and other texts. The web offers an incredible opportunity to become aware of the staggering number of publications that exist in the world **(Fig. 2)**. For a vision institute it is also important to participate actively in the publications in ophthalmology. Articles and chapters in texts produced by our institute colleagues are important elements in maintaining a high level and profile.

Clinical results and the scientific research conducted by the senior surgeon and their team must be collected, analyzed and processed by the statistics department and technical writers. Articles and texts must be written in the correct style, they should be evidence-based and graphs and tables should be employed when presenting quantitative research data.

COOPERATION WITH NATIONAL AND INTERNATIONAL SCIENTIFIC SOCIETIES

There are several international scientific societies in the world dedicated to ophthalmology. The most important are:

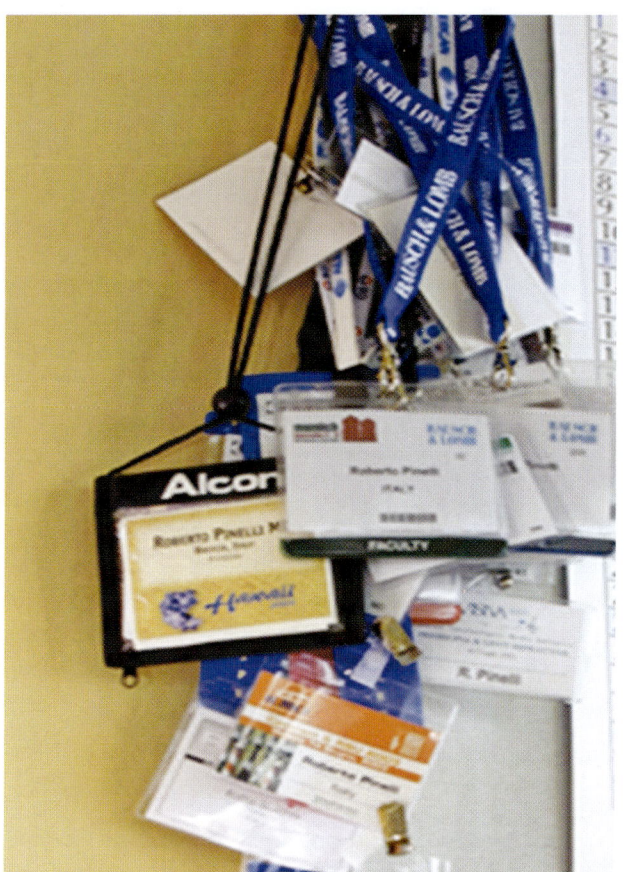

Fig. 2: The most relevant scientific societies organize many international congresses during the year

ASCRS, ESCRS, AAO, ISRS, APAO. In addition, there are the local scientific societies, always of great importance: For Italy there is the SOI (Società Oftalmologica Italiana, which organizes a national and an international symposium every year).

All these scientific societies **(Fig. 3)** organize one or two meetings every year (usually one), which represent occasions of fundamental importance whereby the surgeon and the whole staff of the vision institute can come into direct contact with other situations, services and professionals existing worldwide. This is of key importance because:

- The surgeon can present their clinical results, and also their discoveries and ideas concerning refractive surgery and ophthalmology in general to fellow colleagues at international symposia **(Fig. 4)**. This process of presenting a lecture, or of holding an instructional course as senior

instructor or coinstructor requires thorough and efficient organization in advance. In fact, abstracts usually have to be presented months before the congress, in order to give the scientific committee the opportunity to evaluate them all and choose the most significant. Sometimes the abstract has to be written considering the clinical results that the institute will be able to collect in the following 4-6 months. The typical structure of the abstract can be summarized as follows: Title—Objective/Purpose—Methods—Results —Conclusions. The important thing to keep in mind is that each scientific society has its own rules for writing an abstract (number of words, elements required...). Handouts represent another important aspect to be taken care of in arranging one's participation at a congress. They should be sent to the society some weeks in advance in

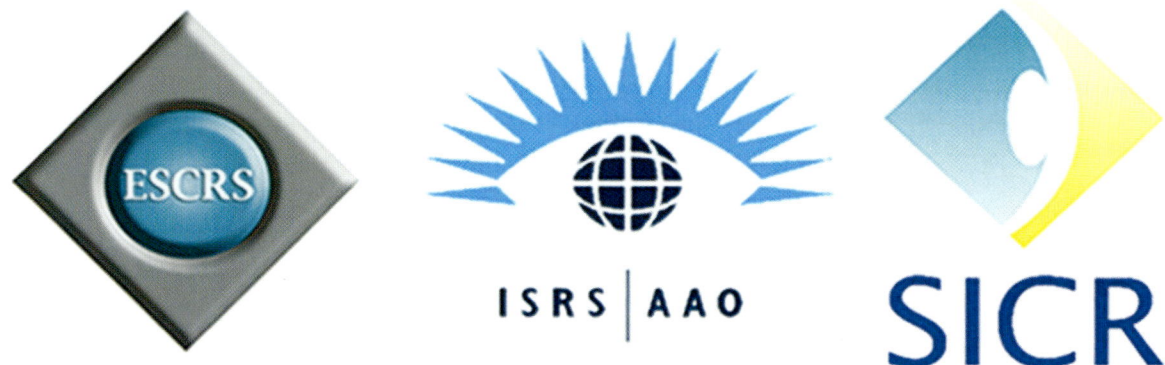

Fig. 3: Some important scientific societies related to refractive surgery

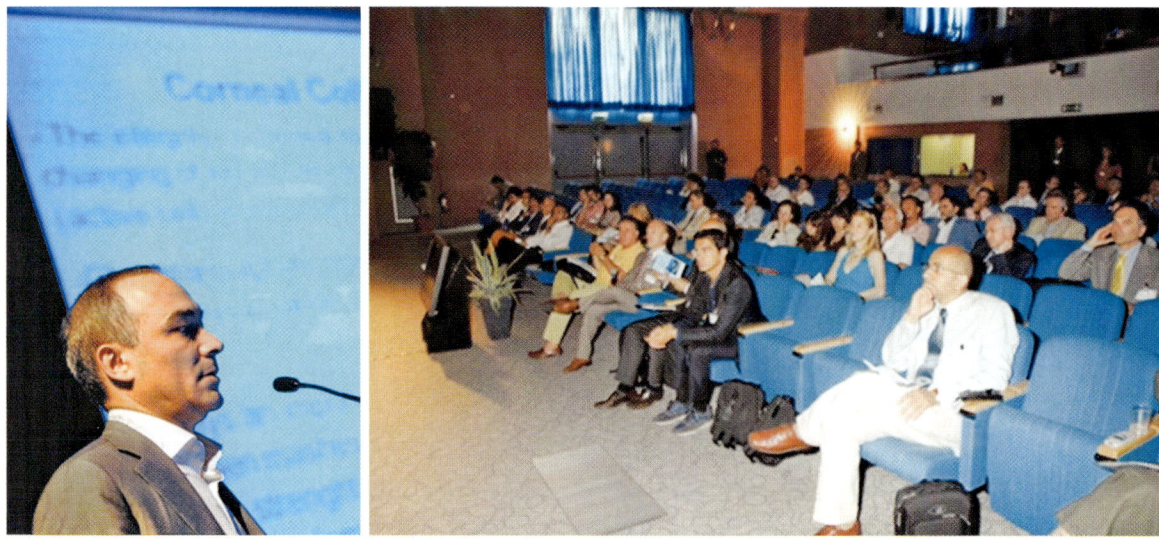

Fig. 4: A session of the 1st World Vision Surgery Symposium in June 2007

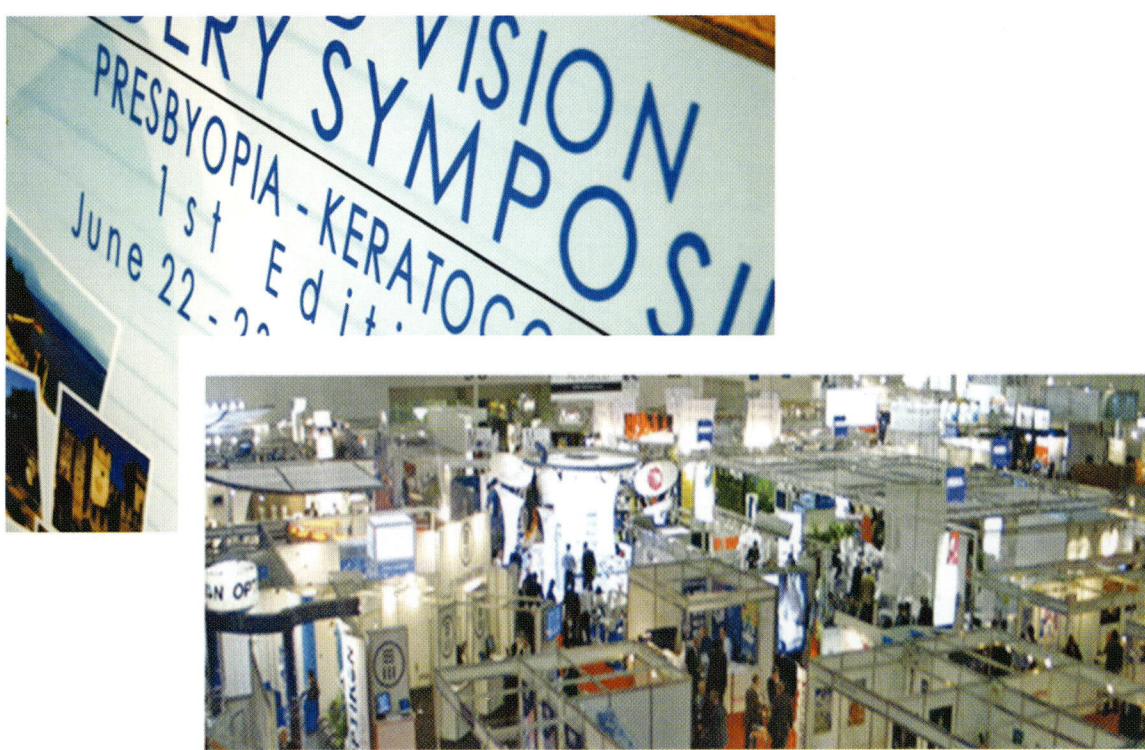

Fig. 5: The preparation of the 1st World Vision Surgery Symposium

order to have them copied and distributed, before, during or after the course attended.

• During these occasions, the surgeon has the chance to attend the colleagues' courses and lectures, comparing his/her results to theirs, with interesting observations.

• At such international events, many companies operating in the main branches of ophthalmology hire booths in the convention centers. This represents an interesting occasion to personally see the newest products on the market all in once place, buying samples of them and finding innovative solutions for the institute at different levels **(Fig. 5)**.

• Furthermore, international congresses represent the best occasion to meet people operating in the field of ophthalmology, leading to fruitful cooperation and forging beautiful friendships, in particular during the cocktails, lunches and dinners organized by the society itself for this very purpose.

CHAPTER 3

Elena Scaffidi

New Operative Tools to Improve the Structure

PSYCHOLOGY OF VISION

Specificity of the Ophthalmic Setting

Is Psychology of Vision a Mere Branch of Experimental Psychology?

It is often popularly believed that psychology of vision is simply a branch of experimental psychology. This is partially true, if we consider that over the last century vision has attracted the interest of psychologists primarily in terms of its functions and the search for correlations between eye and brain.

The eye was at the time considered to be a simple optical instrument, whose function was explicable in terms of cerebral mechanisms **(Fig. 1)**.

Sight is so familiar and apparently so easy that it only takes a little imagination to realize that the eyes, insofar as the visual processes is made possible, pose an extremely difficult problem for the brain to solve.

A series of different paradigms have been proposed to explain the fascinating phenomenon of vision, all ascribable to different theories of perception. The German Herman von Helmholtz (1821–1894), physiologist, physician and psychologist, was the first to describe perceptions as 'unconscious inferences' that link sensory data to external reality. This concept introduces the possibility that a subjective experience could play a significant role in perceiving one's surroundings and that there could be different variables that influence how we think about our visual capacity.

Besides the above huge body of research that has, and still is, being conducted into the perceptual and sensory aspects

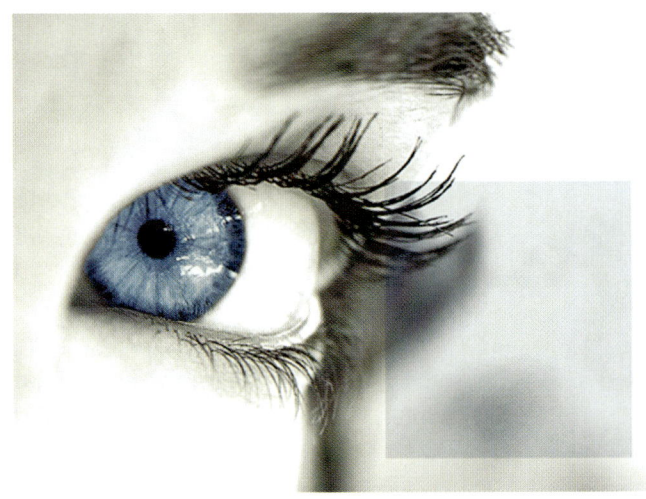

Fig. 1: Psychology of vision is not simply a branch of experimental psychology

of vision, there are nevertheless many other aspects of a psychological nature which cannot avoid being assessed and interpreted in a vision institute where a variety of persons are seen on a daily basis. Along with a vision defect and the desire to correct it, they also bring with them their social background, their culture, their (sometimes unshakeable) certainties, their needs and their fears.

Not to take these aspects into account is tantamount to thinking of the patient as just a pair of eyes and not as a wholly unique individual whose motivations, expectations, and meaning embraced by his decisions within their wider life context may well differ enormously from those of any other individual. In this case we have moved into the area of vision psychology.

What is the Relation between Psyche and Vision?

Vision and mind are strongly connected for different reasons:
- There is a great difference between an objective perception and a subjective perception.
- Different aspects of our daily life use vision to access the symbolic function of individuals to use representations: Memory, dreams, reading, thinking, hearing, music, etc.
- Most people consider vision to be the most important sense, which allows us to move in life and to distinguish persons, events, and behaviors.

That is why when faced with a new patient it is mandatory to proceed with the assessment of subjective dimensions, such as:
- Personality traits (e.g. the obsessive and/or compulsive, depressed, paranoid patient).
- Cognitions (what he was told about his problem and its solutions—other people's experiences, other doctors' advice, etc.).
- Cognitive mechanism (what is the process he most frequently uses to process information and how emotions are integrated with rationality).

- Information (about his visual problem, about surgery, about his own health conditions, about pre- and postoperative phases, etc.).
- Prejudices, stereotypes (influenced by social culture, academic culture, personal history, other people stories, etc.).
- Personal needs, visual needs, relationship needs (important to investigate other aspects of his life to evaluate what he is looking for with surgery).

The above aspects must be examined from a multidisciplinary perspective during the preoperative consultation by all the professionals who meet the patient (OD's, refractive surgeon, nurse). They are then reassessed and confirmed or disconfirmed by the patient counselor during a subsequent interview which is specifically geared towards ensuring that the health professionals are fully aware of these factors—which represent important parameters when assessing the physiological suitability of the patient for surgery—and is also aimed at evaluating the patient's level of information and ascertaining that he has been informed of all the facts regarding his personal visual situation and fully understands the reason why LASIK is considered the best tool to solve his visual problem **(Fig. 2)**.

These skilled professionals have been trained to assess these variables by the vision psychologist who can play an

3 CHAPTER

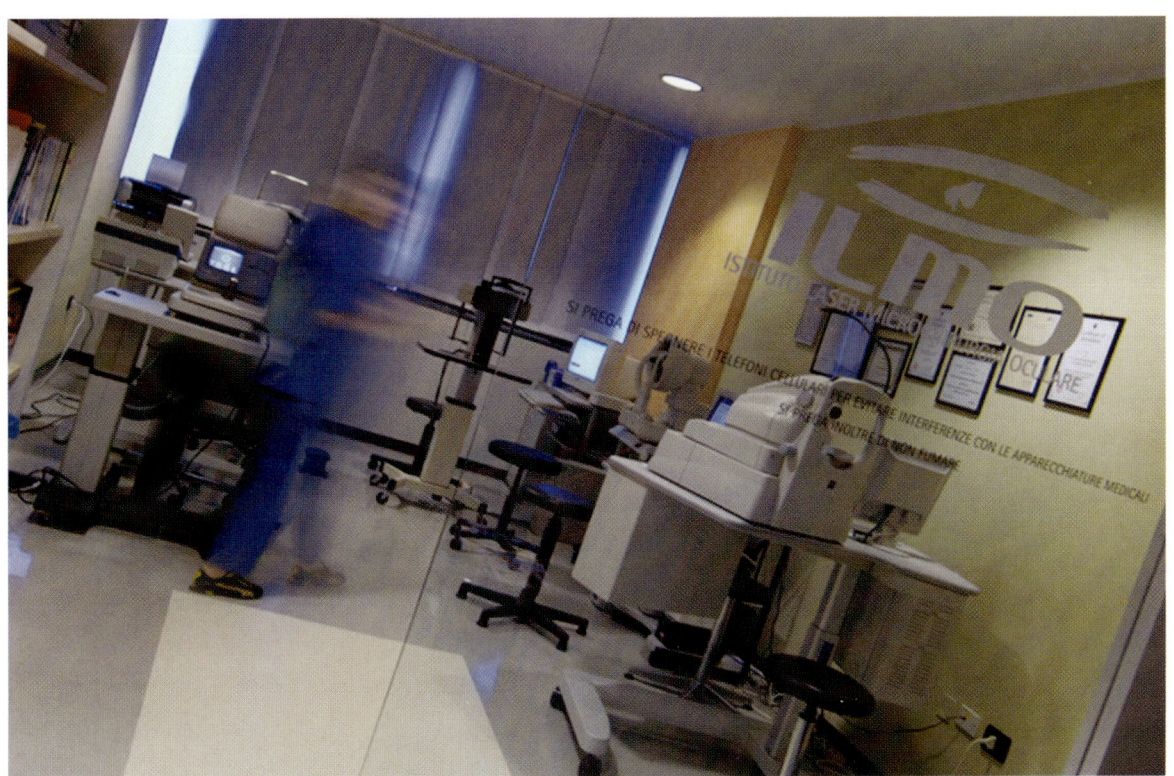

Fig. 2: Diagnostic area

active role in the process of assessment but, more frequently, is to be considered an internal resource, a 'coach' of the personnel.

It is also very important to remember that LASIK surgery is not always mandatory. People can continue to live their own lives wearing glasses or contact lenses. So the gravity of the visual defect can be considered in some cases to demarcate the border line that will justify the patient's asking for surgery.

Does the patient need to undergo surgery?

- Visual impairment can be corrected only with surgery.
- Limitation of subjective feeling of individual potential as a person (at work, within the family environment, with other people, very much linked to self-esteem).
- Patient feels justified in asking for surgery.

Or does he 'simply' desire it?

- How to match the realization of a desire with the feeling of personal responsibility towards the difficult choice to have surgery when it may not be necessary?
- Social support (what do the patient's relatives think about surgery? Do they agree and advise the patient or are they against it?).
- Pros and cons evaluation (risks vs. benefits).
- Is the surgery aimed at solving an aesthetic problem or a functional problem?

The Assessment of Motivation, Expectations and Level of Information

Remember that the patient must be gently interviewed without giving him the impression of being under investigation. He must be offered the chance to speak openly and freely with an expert who is able to answer his questions and provide information that will enable him to arrive at a conscious and mature decision regarding accessing LASIK surgery **(Fig. 3)**.

It can be useful to have an internal checklist of aspects to be verified during the interview with our patient:

- Motivations (why does the patient ask for surgery?).
- Expectations (are they realistic? Does he imagine he will develop 'super-human vision'? What can he really get from surgery and what is beyond the limits of being realistically possible?).
- Level of information (do not give up if the patients seems not to need any information; explain the nature of his vision defect and any differences from other cases/surgical approaches).
- Myths and preconceptions (interview the patient about his family and friends experiences about vision, surgery; lead him to talk about blindness, and try to understand whether he is frightened or concerned, even if he does not openly talk about or express emotions).
- Thoughts and emotions (remember that in human beings what we think is powerfully influenced by what we feel!).

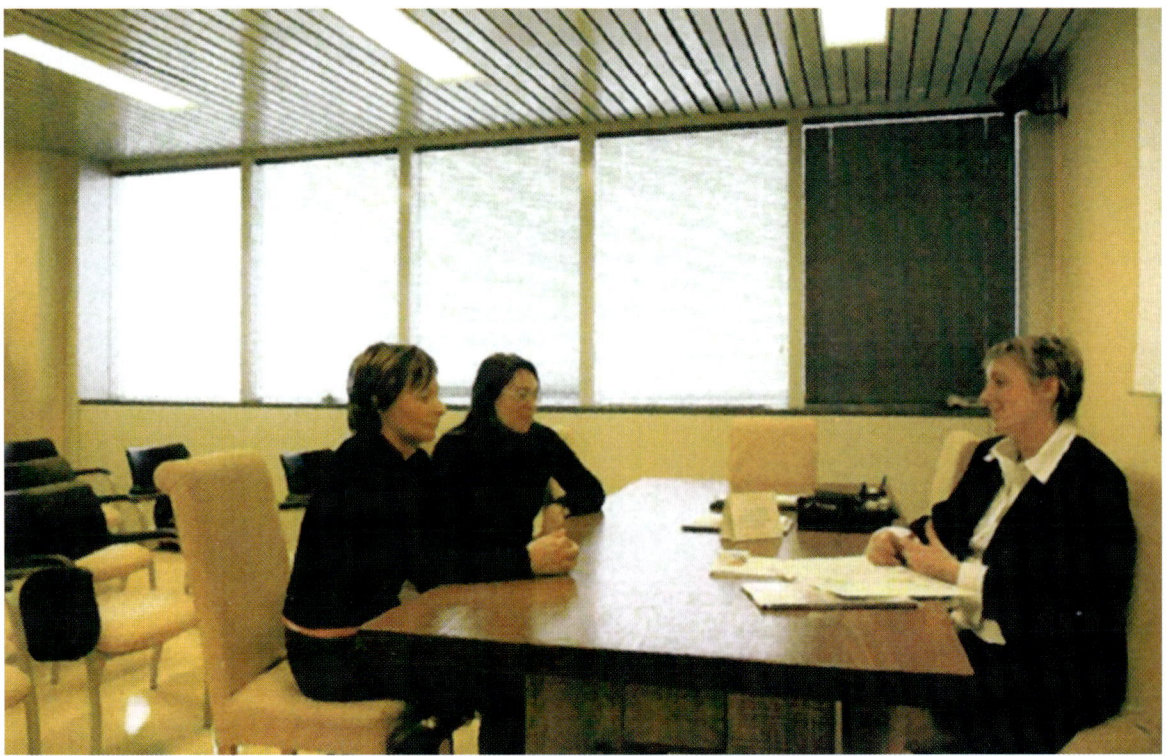

Fig. 3: The first meeting with the patient care

What the Patient Fears and does not have the Courage to Ask?

The above procedure is the first step towards obtaining the patient's informed consent. He knows very well that a document will be given to him before surgery and sometimes he does not exactly understand what it is for. Even though the patient does not ask openly, I believe it is very important to talk to the patient about what informed consent is and what it is not, so that before leaving the ophthalmic center he fully understands that it is a process which provides information and develops awareness in order that he may, of his own free will, decide whether or not to undergo surgery. Furthermore, he should understand that it is not a legal disclaimer merely designed to protect the surgeon. Tell your patient that the surgeon is always responsible for his professional decisions and behaviors, and that any responsibility the surgeon may bear for malpractice would in no way be invalidated by signing the informed consent document **(Fig. 4)**.

The innermost concern of any individual about to embark upon ophthalmic surgery is that of permanently losing his sight. Only some of our patients are able to make this fear explicit, whereas others are socially convinced that is neither appropriate nor elegant to bombard the doctor with questions (after all, the doctor is supposed to be the expert) and also may believe that a direct question could be judged as a psychological weakness on the part of the patient. The reality is that all have the same concern. So do not avoid touching on this point during patient counseling. In addition it will

be necessary to make him aware of the rare, but sometimes possible, inconveniences that can occur during surgery. We need to build a relationship based on mutual respect and trust. For the patient, to understand that his surgeon and the personnel of the institute he has chosen is always open to listen to him and ready to reply to his needs is the best guarantee to foster the patient's trust.

Introducing the Concept of Satisfaction as a Multidimensional Variable

The Evaluation of Satisfaction: What is it for?

Patient satisfaction and quality of life are both patient-centered subjective endpoints. Quality of life depends on medical and psychological factors. Satisfaction with care relies on the different features of the health care received.

Whereas health care managers are long accustomed to patient satisfaction assessment, clinicians are, by contrast, more familiar with the subjective measure of quality of life.

The former are especially concerned with ensuring the competitiveness of the health care service, regarding patient satisfaction data as a marketing tool. The latter are, on the other hand, interested in evaluating the effectiveness of therapies, supplementing this assessment with quality of life data **(Fig. 5)**.

Only recently in clinical research have surgeons also obtained valuable information from patient satisfaction

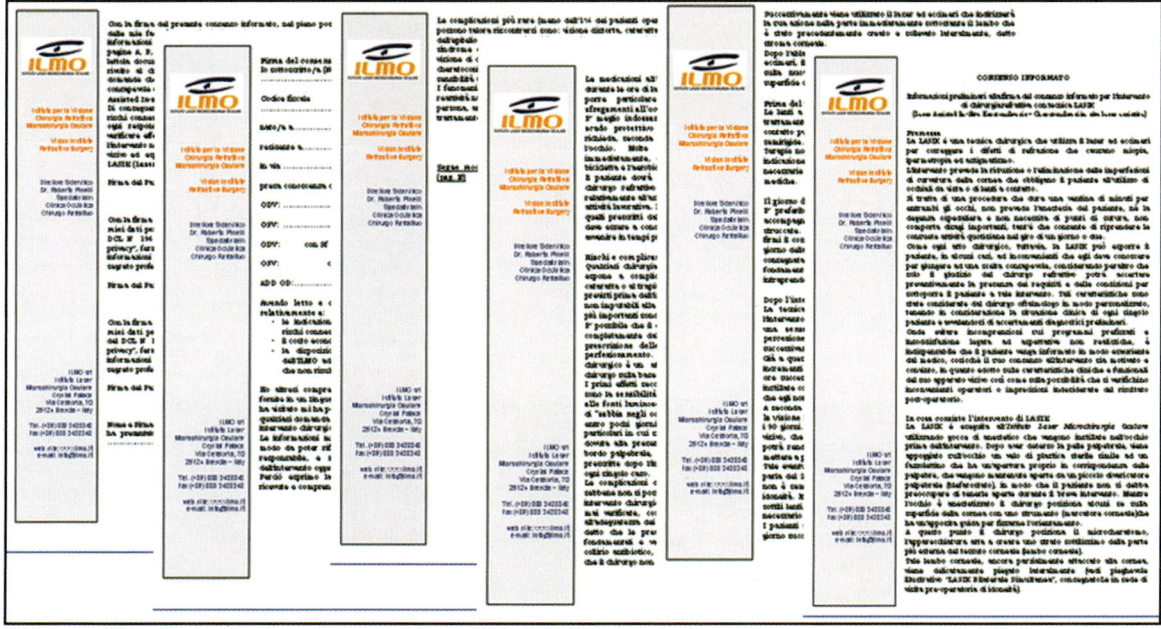

Fig. 4: The patient's informed consent

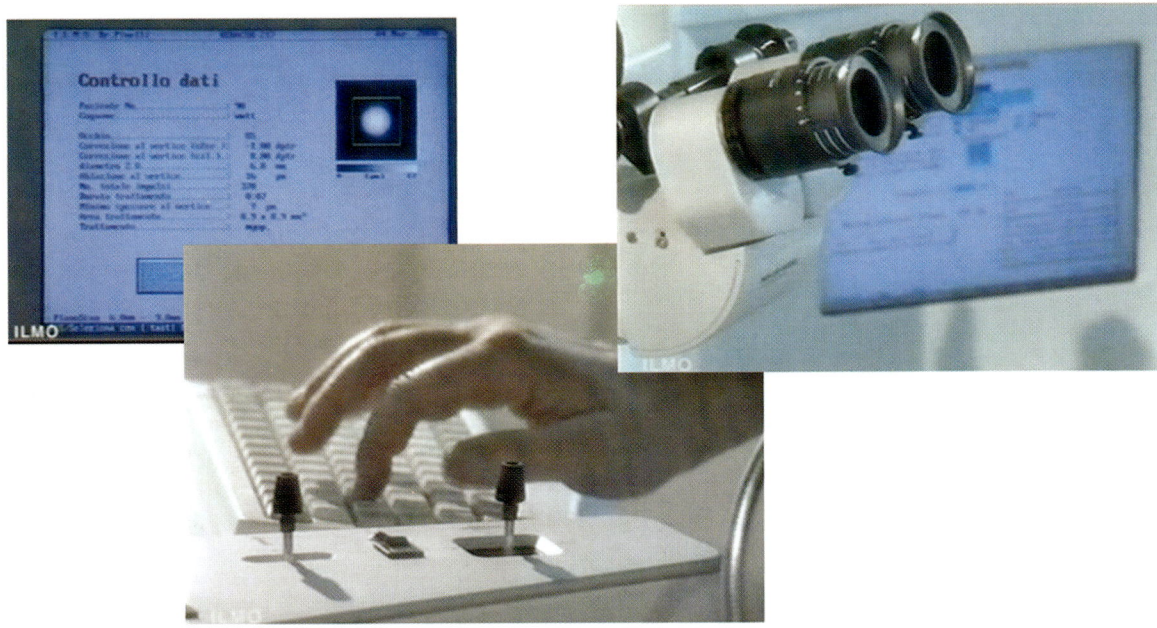

Fig. 5: The evaluation of clinical and patient satisfaction data

assessment. This variable may be viewed as a significant determinant of quality of life.

Patient Satisfaction and Quality of Life Evaluation
Factors involved in patient perception of QoL Medical = type and stage of disease, type of treatment Psychosocial = coping mechanism, family support, socioeconomic status
Factors involved in patient perception of satisfaction Health care received = structure of care, process of care, outcomes

Satisfaction with Surgery = Good Quality of Vision?

In every medical setting exploring the association between patient satisfaction and health-related quality of life is complex. There is not necessarily a unidirectional causal relationship between patient satisfaction and clinical outcome. Patient satisfaction may also be seen as a consequence of improved quality of life or health status.

To this extent, refractive surgery is quite a unique field because it is almost universally acknowledged that a person with a visual defect cannot be considered an ill patient. Also it is no longer controversial that some individuals can perceive themselves as highly damaged by their visual impairment from a functional, aesthetic, behavioral and psychological point of view **(Fig. 6)**.

Thus it is that we find ourselves far more frequently referring to nonpathological patients whose resolution or amelioration of their visual defects can ease their own lives.

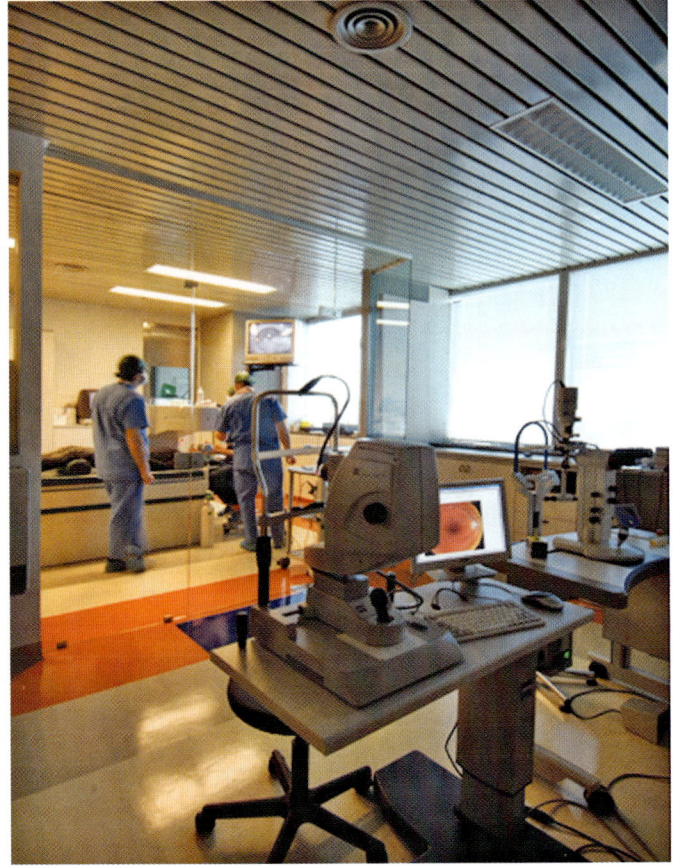

Fig. 6: The laser room

In our comprehensive vision surgery institute we are told on a daily basis of satisfaction for the care received as reported by the patients. Nevertheless we have noticed that some apparent incongruities are still present. For instance, why does an individual with a postoperative outcome who has been assessed as an '8' declare himself happier than does a patient whose postoperative outcomes is rated '10'? This is clear proof that the variables contributing to patient satisfaction personal perception are many and varied.

When refractive surgery developed in Italy about 10 years ago, the initial idea was that LASIK was for people who were not greatly affected by serious ophthalmic disease. In some cases this led ophthalmologists to believe that such patients did not warrant being taken too seriously in their desire to get their needs met together with their visual defects solved. The Italian Refractive Surgery Society in cooperation with the Istituto Laser Microchirurgia Oculare has developed this study with the aim of arriving at a better understanding of those variables which make a patient happy or otherwise and of developing a questionnaire to be administered in different ophthalmic settings to investigate these dimensions **(Fig. 7)**.

One of the purposes of the Italian Refractive Surgery Society is to stress the importance among ophthalmologists of the doctor-patient relationship as an essential tool to comprehend both the visual problem and the person as a whole and to better orientate the doctor's decision-making concerning the surgery technique to be selected.

Patients expectations and needs for health care and also towards refractive surgery are many and varied. The interactions between patients, health professionals, and services are complex. The dependency, uncertainty and anxiety involved in these interactions are likely to influence patients' judgement. It is thus difficult to propose a simple definition of this concept and straightforward criteria for its assessment.

In September 2005 a feasibility, prospective study started within the Istituto Laser Microchirurgia Oculare. In order to define which domains needed to be considered in the questionnaire, we organized three different focus groups led by a psychologist. Both patients who already had already undergone surgery and individuals willing to undergo surgery in the near future took part.

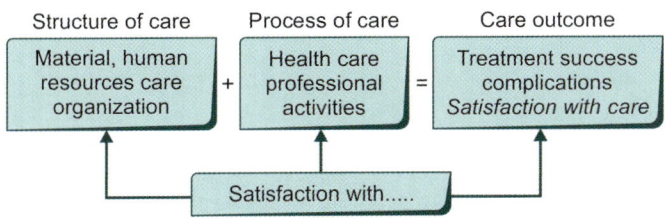

Fig. 7: Patient satisfaction in quality of care assessment in ophthalmology

---

Conceptual Questions Raised in the 3 Focus Groups

- What does patient satisfaction mean?
- What is the relationship between patients' experience, expectations and satisfaction ratings?
- What are the appropriate objects (components) for assessing satisfaction for refractive surgery?
- How much patient comparison between preoperative visual acuity and postoperative outcomes is perceived by patients and what factors can influence their self-perception?

Overlapping Satisfactions: Feedback for the Medical Staff and for the Ophthalmic Administrator

Many patient satisfaction surveys are now performed in medical institutions, mainly in hospitals. Initially, collecting patient satisfaction data may alarm health care providers. It may point out differences in their level of performance. However, these surveys present strategic information for shaping the provision of health care and improving the attractiveness of the institution. As primary witnesses of care, patients may provide valuable perspectives on the performance of the health care institution.

The data they provide through surveys may elicit important suggestions, identify hidden problems and document the impact of efforts made to improve the quality of care **(Fig. 8)**. For example, service quality in health care (waiting times, inconvenience) and in particular, interpersonal aspects of the patient-clinician interactions (unanswered questions, unclear explanations) have been shown to deeply pervade patients' experience of care.

Care outcomes are affected by aspects such as uncertainty regarding the choice of the surgical technique and limited consideration of the patient's overall concerns. Organization managers may focus on these aspects for care improvement and resources allocation.

In clinical practice, patient satisfaction assessment is being increasingly used in assessing consultations and patterns of communication. This evaluation may sensitize clinicians to patient's concerns and allow them to better meet their needs. If shared in the consultation, these data facilitate more effective communication. They may lead to strategies for helping patients to build up more reasonable expectations of care and to promote adherence to, co-operation with treatment by examining reasons for dissatisfaction.

EVALUATION OF PATIENT'S SATISFACTION QUESTIONNAIRE

In December 2005, following the introduction of new surgical technology and the strengthening of international relationships, the Institute decided to embark upon a procedure of surveying and assessing patient satisfaction.

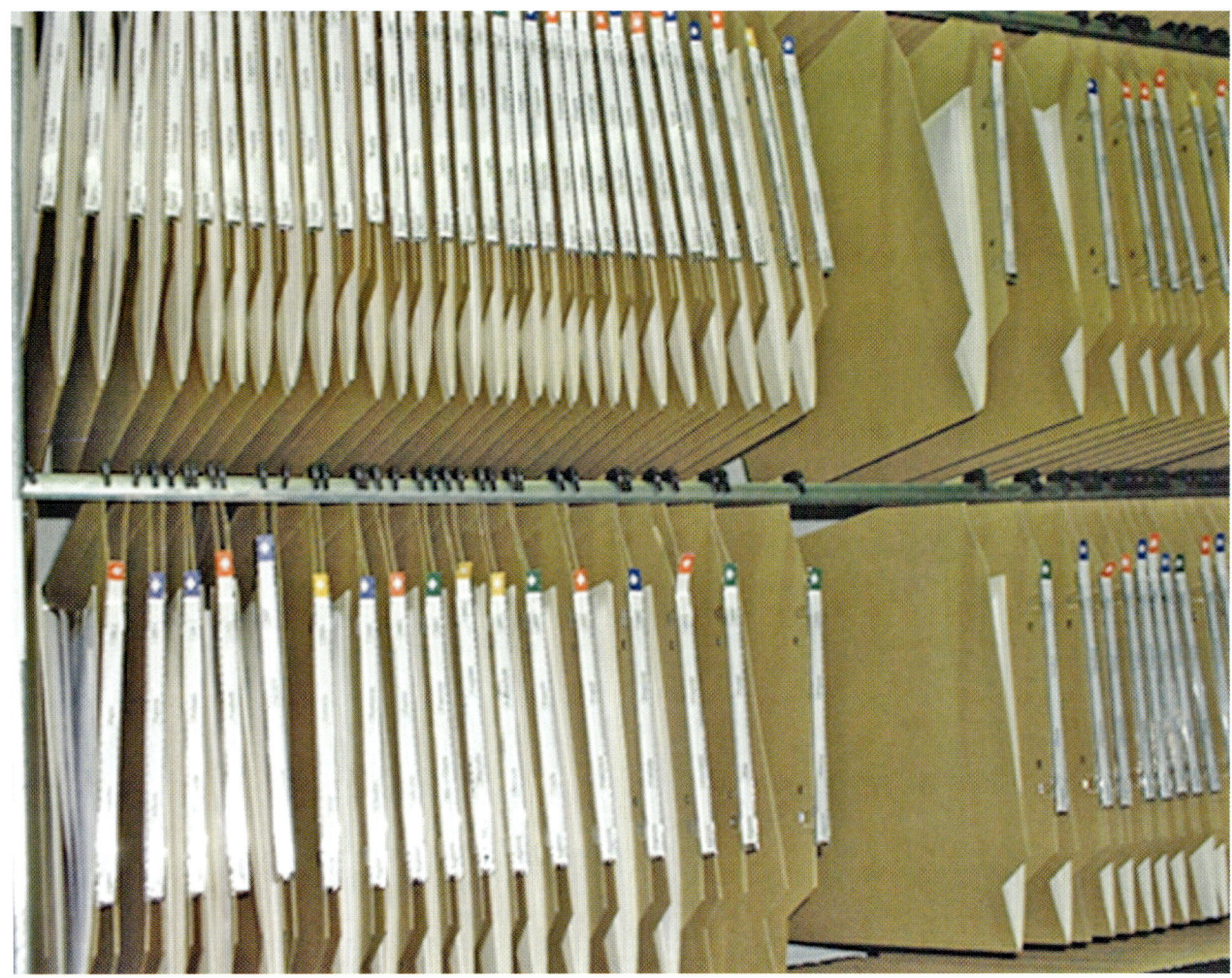

Fig. 8: Clinical folders archive

The psychological aspect of satisfaction comprises a very important part of the evaluating the outcome of refractive surgery, yet it is the most difficult aspect to evaluate in as much as it is not based on measurable or verifiable factors.

The first step was that of setting out the research framework.

Planning a research project involves constructing an overall outline of the investigation to be conducted, which is known as the preliminary framework (**Flow chart 1**). It is essential that when this planning is complete, the desired objectives be clearly set out, the variables of the investigation are defined as precisely as possible, the reference population is specified, the data collecting tools to be used are identified and, if necessary a validation phase of these tools is provided for. The next step is to define a data collection plan, and then process the information collected, calculating the appropriate statistical indexes thereby arriving at a verification of the hypotheses formulated in the preliminary phase.

The analysis concludes with the validation of the tool and the conceptual discussion of the results obtained.

Preliminary Phase: Investigation Objectives

As already indicated, the investigation arose from the requirement of the Institute to assess the level of satisfaction of its patients not exclusively in terms of objective improvement of visual capacity, but also (or indeed especially) taking the more personal factors into consideration, which involved, in addition to surgical outcome, the entire process as experienced by the patients during their period of contact with the Institute.

At the time of planning of the research project the Institute could already boast eight years of direct experience in the field of refractive surgery; furthermore in 2004 the vision psychology unit was inaugurated, and since then it has been dedicated to the exploration and study of all the 'intangibles' linked to the visual process, the approach to surgery and patient satisfaction with the outcome. These two elements proved to be very useful in the problem analysis phase and in defining the objectives.

Flow chart 1: The research project

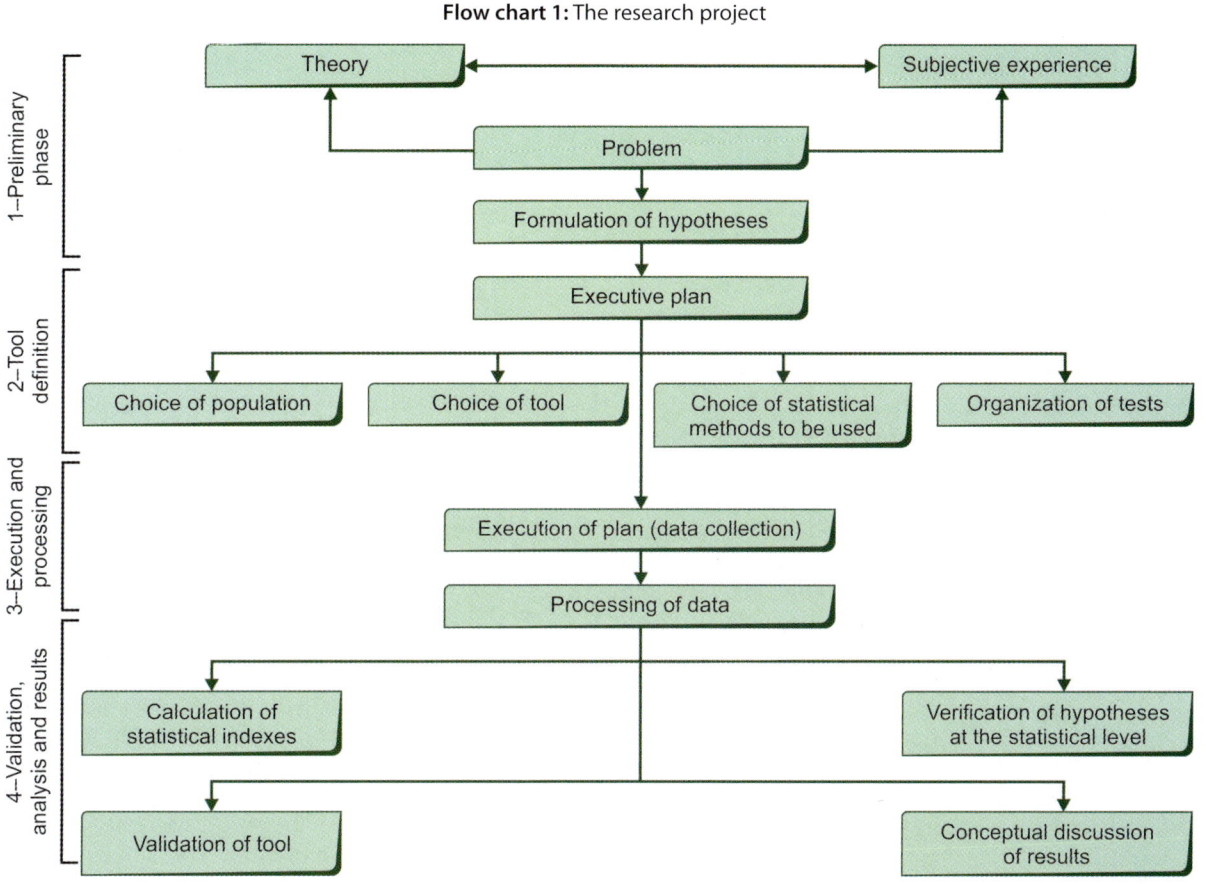

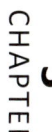

As one may imagine, the analysis of psychological characteristics is beset by a series of difficulties among which are the definition of opinions, attitudes and subjective factors which contribute to such an evaluation. From a statistical point of view this implies the necessity to provide a set of indicators that enable one to evaluate not only extrinsic aspects but also those belonging to the subjective sphere which are of an intrinsic and relational nature. Whereas various models of analysis have been proposed for customer satisfaction, a much-discussed topic in the literature, there has as yet been little discussion regarding patient satisfaction—a decidedly more delicate topic in that it is inherent to health.

Following a long-period of study and reflection on the topic, the Institute identified five aspects for investigation which were considered as offering a good representation of patient satisfaction.

Executive Plan

Population Choice

Initially the investigation was to be conduced only on those patients who were to undergo surgery via the P-curve technique. At the request of the medical area and the vision

psychology unit, the institute decided to broaden its study to include all of its patients. This choice undoubtedly called for greater effort on the part of the institute in that the number of persons involved in the survey was significantly increased and different responses on the basis of the different possible situations had to be provided for, but at the end of the survey this proved to be an optimal situation since it enabled the institute to possess a complete overview of the opinions of its patients, providing the possibility to examine the satisfaction of patients who had undergone different techniques.

Choice of Tools and their Definition

Having determined the study population, it is necessary to define the investigation tools. Some of the factors influencing their choice were:
- The need to request direct opinions regarding institute staff
- Time required to conduct the investigation (period following the operation and differing according to the type of operation)
- Administration of a high number of persons
- The need to leave an appropriate period of time for the patient to respond without pressure, yet at the same time, attempting to avoid distractions.

Taking all these factors into consideration, the vision psychology service, together with the biostatistics unit favored the use of the self-administered questionnaire, which was handed to every patient at the conclusion of their check-up examination.

A fundamental role is carried out by the patient care staff in that they have to present the survey to the patient, explain its objectives and how to complete it, and, having handed it to the patient, being available should any clarifications or explanations be needed.

As indicated, since the questionnaire had to be calibrated against different surgical techniques, the fact that these techniques required differing postoperative adjustment periods had to be taken into consideration. For this reason it was necessary to allow different timing pathways on the basis of each postoperative procedure. At the same time as the first check-up the full questionnaire was administered containing questions regarding personal data, reasons behind the choice to undergo the operation, in which institute and using which technique, satisfaction with treatment, and any pain felt during or after the operation. Subsequently, at the 3, 6 and 12 months check-up the patient again went through just the series of items related to assessment of visual adjustment and satisfaction with the outcome of the intervention.

Statistical Methods

We have already indicated that, satisfaction being a latent variable, we needed to find subjective indicators which, appropriately combined, would enable us to arrive at the variable which was the object of the investigation.

These subjective indicators were created with the ultimate aim of supplying valid and reliable measures which could then be used in models of varying complexity for the verification of our theoretical hypotheses.

The following two phases may be distinguished:
1. The determination of a group of $m > p$ simple indicators $q' = (q_1, q_2, ..., q_m)$, which are assumed to be in relation with the latent variables.
2. The adoption of an $f(q)$ procedure which enables a p-dimensional compound indicator $x' = (x_1, x_2, ..., x_p)$ to be constructed to be used as a scale for measuring latent variables.

In phase 1 the data were collected by inserting into the questionnaire numerous questions assumed to be in some way connected with the constructs of interest; the replies to such questions were inserted into scales with ordered categories which expressed the level of agreement, for example from 'not at all satisfied' to 'very satisfied'. With a view to statistical analysis these categories were represented by means of a numerical code (from 1 to 5 or 7); the quantification of each observed variable represented a simple indicator of the latent variables. In phase 2 it is common practice to construct a compound indicator, which

is associated with p latent variables, using the sum of the m simple indicators.

$$x = f(q) = \sum_{j=1}^{m} a_j q_j \text{ with weightings } a_j' = (a_{j1}, a_{j2}, ..., a_{jp})$$

It is important to remember that the synthesis carried out via compound indicators is not equivalent to the latent variable but represents only the empirical and operational version, that is to say an estimate whose reliability should be evaluated on a case by case basis with the available data. The employment of a relatively large number of simple indicators can at least in part reduce the problems deriving from the fact that subjects have a tendency to give replies which suffer from a certain margin of inaccuracy. This may also be desirable should the questions happen to touch on topics of a somewhat delicate nature. The weightings to be assigned at the indicator construction phase are estimated by means of appropriate statistical procedures together with considerations regarding methodology and robustness of results.

With reference to the properties of the q simple indicators constructed on the basis of observed responses on ordinal scales, it is necessary that every item and the related response scale be interpreted in a basically analogous manner by the subjects; this assumption requires that the phrasing of questions be simple and clear. Even if the condition of homogeneity is met, the ordinal nature of the responses however, does not permit the property of linearity of variables to be attributed *a priori*: in other words one cannot assume that numbers 1, 2, ... (representative of response categories) are equidistant. For this reason, when ordinal variables are available it is good practice to employ models that do not assume linearity of ordinal variables *a priori* and to then verify whether such a restriction is plausible for the data one has available.

For the patient satisfaction study the Institute decided to adopt the algorithmic model of 'Non-linear Principal Component Analysis' (NLPCA), which enables one to distinguish between subjects as clearly as possible. The model enables the determination of the combination of weights that maximizes such separation; from a statistical point of view this means choosing the weights a_j that, if the simple indicators q are fixed, enable one to obtain the maximum variance for each of the p components of x.

Four Macroareas of the Investigation and the Definition of the Single Item

In the light of all the observations made, the Institute decided to divide the questionnaire into four sections:
1. Personal section
2. General information
3. Intervention and recovery
4. Satisfaction.

The entire Institute staff was involved in defining the single items. Each staff member was requested to identify certain aspects which in their opinion were fundamental for assessing the patient in their particular field. For example, the medical area was assigned the task of determining the scales for evaluation of long and near visual capacity. Once the questionnaire had been created a training session was organized in which the staff underwent the final version of the questionnaire, during which they were able to discuss further the formulation of certain questions and the method of administering the questionnaire to patients.

Personal section: The questionnaire is not anonymous since it is necessary for the Institute to be able to compare, at the results analysis stage, patient satisfaction and patient perception of outcome with the medical data contained in the patient medical record.

General information: The questions in this section serve to highlight the sources of information regarding refractive surgery, why the patient decided to undergo the operation, the patient's visual defect, and the main reason for which the patient opted for the technique that was performed.

Intervention and recovery: This section is in fact divided into two: The intervention itself and post-intervention. Regarding the former, the patient is asked to provide their opinion regarding the information given him by the surgeon and surgical staff concerning the operation and everything associated with it. The patient is then asked to evaluate his visual capacity before the intervention, the level he hoped to reach after surgery, and his current visual capacity. The second part is designed to find out whether the patient experienced any problems after surgery, whether he felt any discomfort or pain, and the time taken for his vision to stabilize after surgery. In addition he is asked if he needed a second operation in one or both eyes in order to perfect the results obtained in the first operation and whether he considers that the outcome of the operation corresponds with the information he received during the preoperative examination.

Satisfaction: This is obviously the central part of the questionnaire in which the patient is asked, more or less directly, to express various opinions concerning his degree of satisfaction with different aspects.

The composite indicators determined refer to:
- Technical and professional quality
- Interpersonal relations and communicative abilities
- Internal organization of the Institute
- Surroundings.

For each of these, several simple indicators were determined (from 3 to 8 per composite), on which the patient had to express an opinion ranging from 1–very dissatisfied to 7–very satisfied.

For example:

1. Please state your level of satisfaction regarding *Technical and professional quality*	Very dissatisfied					Very satisfied	
• The manner in which diagnostic examinations were conducted	1	2	3	4	5	6	7
• Competence of doctors	1	2	3	4	5	6	7
• Competence of assistants (orthoptist, optician, operating theater technician	1	2	3	4	5	6	7

Another aspect to be studied concerned the patient's perception of quality of life following the intervention. Quality of life being difficult to define in as much as it is a latent construct, several simple indicators were determined, among which were degree of worry regarding visual deficit, the necessity to ask others for help, and how this aspect was influenced by the surgery.

Validation

At this point, it was necessary to validate the questionnaire we had created for the survey. In fact, independently of the measuring scale used or the characteristic being measured it is necessary to demonstrate that the tool being used for research is valid, i.e. it effectively measures the variable. The concept of validity of psychological measurements often depends on the theory underlying the construction of the tool: if the theory is not completely shared, the tests one uses may be differently valid or differ in certain aspects.

In addition to being valid, the tool must also be reliable: The measurement that we take today regarding a certain characteristic should, all conditions being equal, be substantially analogous to that which we take at a later time. Summarizing, a psychometric tool should therefore be:
- Objective
- Sensitive and discriminating
- Reliable and consistent
- Valid.

By validity of content is meant the capacity to accurately represent the whole gamut of possible behaviors linked to the psychological characteristic one intends to measure; usually this is based on the opinion of experts and does not need statistical concepts. When one refers to conceptual validity one must demonstrate the extent to which the performance of the test in relation to the construct one wishes to measure, using for example factorial analysis, multivariate analysis of variance and multiple regression.

To verify our tool we provided for its validation phase, inserting a battery of questions at the end of the questionnaire aimed precisely at the above-mentioned aspects and at highlighting any problems or difficulties the patient might have encountered in the compilation phase **(Fig. 9)**.

The assessment section is repeated at the end of each compilation so as to evaluate the tool during the process of its administration.

Execution

Data Collection

As mentioned earlier, it is the patient care team that occupies the main role in this phase, and administers the questionnaire directly to the patient. The manner in which the patient deals with the survey the consequent quality of their responses may also depend on the way in which they are involved in it. It is therefore essential that there be someone present who will explain the objectives of the survey to them and who will make themselves available to answer any queries and, if necessary, encourage the patient to complete the questionnaire accurately and fully.

Data Processing

In order to analyze the data a database was created to meet the needs determined at the questionnaire preparation and statistical model decision making phase.

The initial phase of data collection lasted three months, at the end of which we started to process the information obtained from the patients.

The number of questionnaires from the initial administering (those handed out to the patients at their first postoperative check-up) was such as to enable a complete analysis to be undertaken along with a first revision of the questionnaire. The number of questionnaires returned from the second administering was, on the other hand, insufficient to proceed (the first time limit before readministration was in fact three months).

The first step was that of conducting a clean-up operation of the data itself and verifying the data coherence. Usually this is a somewhat delicate process in that the database must be handled directly to manage any input errors or those arising from any lack of understanding (albeit involuntary) on the part of the respondent. It is at this point that a decision must be taken concerning how to handle missing data. The first thing we noticed was that the percentage of missing data was indeed very low, i.e. almost all patients answered all the questions completely. This was probably because the patients felt involved in the survey and understood the reasons for it when it was presented to them by the patient care staff.

Once the data clean-up operation had been carried out, data analysis was conducted, the results being differentiated according to the surgical technique of reference. First all, descriptive analyzes were performed referring to the reference population (sex, age and profession), represented by means of simple histograms. The statistical model was then applied (Non-linear Principal Component Analysis). The results were

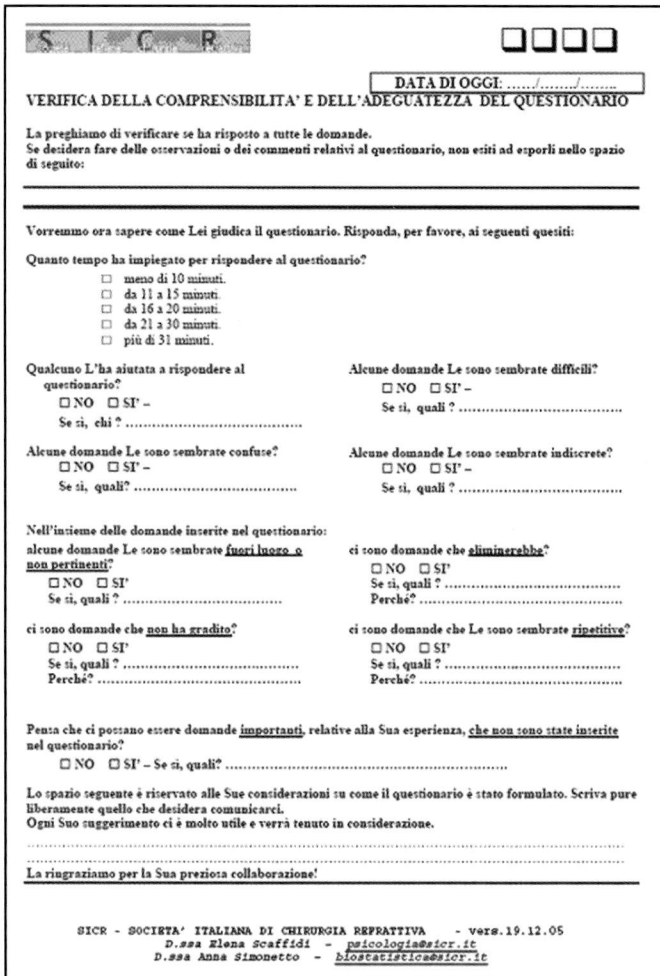

Fig. 9: Verification of the comprehension and adequacy questionnaire

surprising. For example the overall average satisfaction was equivalent to 8 (1 = not at all satisfied, scale 1 and 10 = very satisfied).

At the end of the data processing period, the questionnaire validation procedure was carried out. This took into account the problems encountered during the clean-up and coherence verification phase, the results obtained from processing and the information contained in that part of the questionnaire dedicated to its own validation. Essentially, two problems were found: one concerning the question regarding the patient's perception of pain, and the other regarding the length of the questionnaire itself. Regarding the first, it was noticed that a considerable percentage of patients who underwent a particular technique reported slight pain/discomfort during and immediately after the operation. This came as a surprise to many, since in the experience of the Institute a characteristic of the technique is that that it does not cause the patient pain. After a brief meeting with the medical area and vision psychology staff, it was concluded that the respondents could have been misled by the fact that the question asks "Did you feel sensations of discomfort or pain?", and does not differentiate between pain and discomfort which are in fact two substantially different aspects. It is very important, in fact, to know if a respondent has simply felt slight discomfort (obviously due to the fact that they have undergone an eye operation), or if they have really felt actual pain. To resolve this question, steps were taken to distinguish between the two aspects in the questionnaire, asking first of all if the patient felt discomfort and then asking if they had felt pain.

Concerning the fact that some considered the number of questions to be too high, we asked ourselves whether all the questions included were relevant in terms of the aims of the investigation. However the statistical model employed used all the variables included, attributing a significant importance to each one. This, plus the fact that despite commenting on the excessive length of the questionnaire, practically all the patients completed it carefully and in full, led us to decide not to change it. It might, however, be useful to let the patients know right from the start how much time is needed to complete the questionnaire.

BIBLIOGRAPHY

1. Baker R. Development of a questionnaire to assess patients' satisfaction with consultations in general practice. British Journal of General Practice. 1990;40(341):487-90.
2. Bernhart MH, Wiadnyana IGP, Wihardjo H, et al. Patient satisfaction in developing countries. Social Science and Medicine. 1999;48:989-96.
3. Calnan M, Katsouyiannoupoulos V, Ovcharov VK, Proshorskas R, Ramic H, Williams S. Major determinants of consumer satisfaction with primary care in different health systems. Family Practice. 1994;11:468-78.
4. Gasquet I. Satisfaction des patients et performance hospitalière. La Presse Médicale. 1999;28:1610-16.
5. Gregory RL. Eye and Brain. Raffaello Cortina Editore, 1998.
6. Rubin HR, Ware JE, Nelson EC, et al. The Patient Judgement of Hospital Quality (PJHQ) questionnaire. Medical Care. 1990;28:S17-S18.
7. Sitzia J, Wood N. Patient satisfaction: A review of issues and concepts. Social Science and Medicine. 1997;45:1829-43.
8. Ware JE, Snyder MK, Wright WR, et al. Defining and measuring patient satisfaction with medical care. Evaluation and Program Planning. 1983;6:247-63.

3 CHAPTER

SECTION 2

Overview

CHAPTER 4

Tangwa Martin Neville

Eye Aberrations: Overview

CLINICAL CONTROLLER—ISTITUTO LASER MICROCHIRURGIA OCULARE

When a light point or source emanates light, it travels in rays in different directions[1,31-34]—Parallel rays travelling in a given direction may hit a surface and are either reflected absorbed or transmitted. When the surface is an optical surface it will either converge the rays to form an image or diverge the same to a second plain to form a virtual image. Geometrical optics describes this behavior in a series of laws.[7-11]

Optical systems produce images emanating from sources, objects, light points and the visual world by converging or diverging the rays to focal points. A wavefront is a surface over which an optical disturbance forms, and is in constant phase and normal to the light rays.[16-18]

The eye is an optical system that conveys the visual world to the retina. Thus, light coming from a point source or object will be conveyed to the retina through the pupil and the refracting surfaces; the main being the cornea and crystalline lens.[2-16] Others include the aqueous humor, vitreous humor and the tear film. The complexity of the system is quite clear. It is well-known that the eye is not a perfect optical system. In a perfect or emmetropic eye the resulting wavefront would be a flat wavefront, i.e. without impurities or aberrations. This flat wavefront is known as the piston or reference. In the eye the rays converge at different image points from this ideal, and the distance measured in microns is the wavefront aberration.[2-10]

Principally, the aberrations in the eye are determined by the disalignment of it's main optical elements the cornea and the crystalline lens with the visual axis.[2-13] Other elements are the state of the tear film the vitreous and aqueous humor

eventual scars from surgery, trauma and disease. Aberrations however change and increase with age.[9-24] Of great clinical importance is the pupil diameter, it has been estimated that the best functional diameter would be 3–3.2 mm; the wider the pupil the more disturbing the aberrations are, while smaller pupils lead to diffraction which also disturbs image quality.

Eye aberrations are classified into low and higher order and are generally studied at the pupil area.[8-20] They have been graded mathematically using the Zernike polynomial expansions, which can describe an infinite number of aberrations and of the 60 sorted out thus far, eye scientists use the first 15 as it is understood that these can completely describe the visual scenery. In the Zernike polynomials the superscript describes the angular frequency; the number of times the wavefront repeats itself while the subscript describes the order.[16-19] On this basis and with this name a triangle of aberrations and list of modes have been designed **(Figs 1A and B)**.

The low order aberrations which form 80–90% of the total, start off at the zero aberration or piston which is the reference point. It is flat, the first order aberration tilt or prism is also of no clinical importance.[7]

Very familiar to the ophthalmologists are the second order aberrations—defocus or visual defects myopia, hyperopia, presbyopia and symmetrical astigmatism. These are the daily refractive defects corrected with spectacle glasses, contact lenses and more often today with refractive surgery. They cause visual blurring, loss of visual lines and management has thus far been efficient safe and of great patient appreciation.

Higher order aberrations make up 10–17% of the total aberrations. These have more complex geomertical forms,

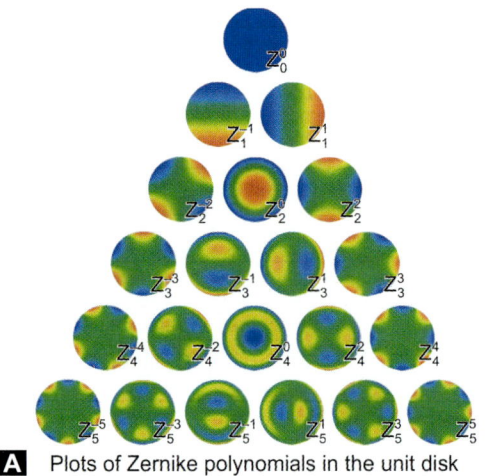

A   Plots of Zernike polynomials in the unit disk

Zernike term	Name
Z_0^0	Piston
Z_1^1, Z_1^{-1}	Tilt (Prism)
Z_2^0	Defocus
Z_2^2, Z_2^{-2}	Astigmatism
Z_4^2, Z_4^{-2}	Secondary astigmatism
Z_4^0	Spherical aberration
Z_3^1, Z_3^{-1}	Coma
Z_3^3, Z_3^{-3}	Trefoil
Z_4^4, Z_4^{-4}	Quatrefoil

B

Figs 1A and B: (A) Zernike images; (B) Zernike classification

cause difficulties like haloes, glare, ghost images starburst patterns and diplopia especially in low lighting conditions and during night driving, third order aberrations are Coma and trefoil. Trefoil is an aberration of little clinical significance.[28]

Coma is present in keratoconus, decentered corneal grafts, intraocular lenses and laser ablations; as well as in asymmetric astigmatism.[8-11] It has a comet graphic shape, is highly influenced by pupil diameter, causes reduction in visual lines, ghost images haze polydiplopia.

Fourth order aberrations are secondary astigmatism, quadrafoils of little clinical significance[20] and spherical aberration. This aberration is spherical in shape with the graphic form of a Mexican hat the sombrero. It causes loss of contrast sensitivity, haloes and night myopia, could increase after myopic lasik.[12-30] Most wave aberration depends on second order aberrations which have a square radius dependency, such that the increase in overall wave aberration with pupil size is reported to increase approximately by the second power of the pupil diameter. The normal human eye has some amount of spherical aberration, which is positive for about one diopter in mydriasis. It is dependent on pupil diameter and the wavelength of incident light. The longitudinal spherical aberration is positive for the cornea and negative for the crystalline and young accommodating lens.[15-30] While in the positive aberration-undercorrected, the marginal rays go to focus before the axial and paraxial rays, in the negative, hypercorrected, which is of the crystalline lens the axial and paraxial rays are first in focus. The energy distribution to the photoreceptors scales down from the peripheral rays to the central so that the eye downgrades the images formed, by high lighting those conveyed by the axial and paraxial rays. The same holds for the directionality of retinal receptors and the Stiles-Crawford phenomenon.

The pentafoils, secondary trefoils, coma are other higher order aberrations which do not cause clinically significant problems. Higher order aberrations are useful in as much as they are capable and responsible for countering chromatic aberrations.[22,23] In the era of refractive surgery it is believed and to some extent some of these aberrations are already being treated.through customized ablations.

REFERENCES

1. Applegate RA, Thibos LN, Hilmantel G. Optics of aberroscopy and supervision. Journal of Cataract and Refractive Surgery. 2001;27(7):1093-107.
2. Artal P, Guirao A. Contributions of the cornea and the lens to the aberrations of the human eye. Optic Letters. 1998;23:1713-5.
3. Artal P, Berrio E, Guirao A, Piers P. Contribution of the cornea and internal surfaces to the change of oculare aberrations with age. J Opt Am A. 2002:137-43.
4. Atchison D, Collins M, Wildsoet C, Christensen J, Waterworth M. Measurement of monochromatic aberrations of human eyes as a function of accomodation by the Howland aberroscope technique. Vis Res. 1995;35:313-23.
5. Atchinson D, Smith G. Schematic eyes. In: Atchinson D Smith G (Eds). Optics of the Human Eye. London Butterworth-Heinemann; 2000: Appendix 3.
6. Barbero S, Marcos S, Merayo-Lloves JM. Total and corneal aberrations in an unilateral aphakic subject. J cat Refract Surg. 2002;28:1594-1600.
7. Born M, Wolf E. Principles of optics (6th edn) Pergamon Press, Oxford 1993.
8. Buhren J, Kuhne C, Kohnen T. Defining subclinical keratoconus using corneal first-surface higher-order aberrations. Am J opthalmol. 2007;143:3424-32.
9. Castejon-Mochon FJ, Lopez-Gil N, Benito A, Artal P. Oculare wave-front aberration statistics in a normal young population. Vis Res. 2002;42:926-36.
10. Charman WN, Jennings JAM. Objective measurments of the longitudinal chromatic aberration of the human eye. Vis Res. 1976;16:999-1005.
11. Charman WN. The optics of the eye. In: Bass M (Ed). Handbook of optics (2nd edn) Mcgraw-Hill, New York (NY) 1995.

12. Collins MJ, Wildsoet CF, Atchinson DA. Monochromatic aberrations and myopia. Vis Res. 1995;35:1157-63.

13. Guirao A, Artal P. Off-axis monochromatic aberrations estimated from double pass easurements in the human eye. Vis Res. 199;39:207-17.

14. He JC, Marcos S, Webb RH, Burns SA. Measurement of the wave-front aberration of the eye by a fast psychophysical procedure. J Opt Soc Am A. 1998;15:2449-54.

15. He JC, Burns SA, Marcos S. Monochromatic aberrations in the accomodated human eye. Vis Res. 2000;200:41-8.

16. Hofer H, Artal P, singer B, Aragon J, Williams D. Dynamics of the human eye wave aberration. J Opt Soc Am A. 2001;18:497-506.

17. Jennings JAM, Charman WN. Off-axis image quality in the human eye. Vis Res. 1981;21:445-55.

18. Lombardo M, Lombardo G. Wave aberration of human eyes and new descriptors of image optical quality and visual performance. Journal of cataract and refractive surgery. 2010;36(2):313-31.

19. Myron Yanoff, Jay S Duker. Opthalmology (3rd edn) Mosby Elsevier. 2009.

20. Mahajan VN. Zernike circle polynomials and optical aberrations of systems with circular pupil. Appl Opt. 1994;38:8121-4.

21. Marcos S, Burns SA. On the symmetry between eyes of wavefront aberration and cone directionality. Vis Res. 2000;40: 2437-47.

22. Marcos S, Burns SA, Moreno-Barriuso E, Navarro R. A new approach to the study of ocular chromatic aberrations. Vis Res. 1999;39:4309-23.

23. Mclellan JS, Marcos S, Prieto PM, Burns SA. Imperfect Optics may be the eye's defence against chromatic blur. Nature. 2002; 17:696-9.

24. Mclellan J, Marcos S, Burns S. Age related changes in monochromatic wave aberrations in human eyes. Invest Ophalmol Vis Sci. 2001;42:1390-5.

25. Navarro R, Artal R, Williams DR. Modulation transfer of the human eye as a function of retinal eccentricity. J Opt Soc Am A. 1993;10:201-12.

26. Navarro R, Moreno E, Dorronsoro C. Monochromatic aberrations and point spread functions of the human eye across the visual field. J Opt Soc Am A. 1998;15:2522-9.

27. Porter J, Guirao A, Cox I, Williams D. Monochromatic aberrations of the human eye in a large population. J opt Soc Am A. 2001;18:1793-1803.

28. Rapuano Christopher J. American Academy of Ophthalmology, Basic and clinical science course section 13: refractive surgery. 2011.

29. Rynders MC, Lidkea BA, Chisholm WJ, Thibos LN, Haggerty KM. Distribution of pupil centers with respect to the visual axis. Optometry and vision science. 1993;70:157-8.

30. Rynders MC, Navarro R, Losada MA. Objective measurment of the off-axis longitudinal chromatic aberration in the human eye. Vis Res. 1998;38:513-22.

31. Seiler T, Kaemmerer M, Mierdel P, Krinke HE. Ocular optical aberrations after refractive keratectomy for myopia and myopic astigmatism. Arch Opthalmol. 2000;11817-21.

32. Simonet P, Campbell MCW. The optical transvers chromatic aberration on the fovea of the human eye. Vis Res. 1990;30:187-206.

33. Thibos LN, Bradley A, Still DL, Zhang X, Howarth PA. Theory and measurement of ocular chromatic aberration. Vis Res. 1990;30:33-49.

34. Wang L, Santella RM, Booth M, Kock DD. Higher order aberrations from the internal optics of the eye. J cataract Refract. Surg. 2005;1512-9.

CHAPTER **4**

CHAPTER 5

Jesús Andrés Rosas Apráez, Juan Pablo Castañeda Borrero, Luis Antonio Ruiz

An Approach to the Wavefront Technology: Aberrometry Basis

OVERVIEW AND HISTORY

A new trend breaks in the field of refractive surgery and the study of visual quality: the study of wavefront or aberrometry, a science very new for us, eye care professionals, but since mid-seventies it sat his important start from the astrophysical scientific concerns about improving the images of celestial objects captured by their telescopes. The atmosphere, gaseous layer surrounding our planet, is composed of different gases densities. When the image of a celestial object crosses from vacuum of space different densities of atmospheric gases, the image captured by telescopes deforms and distorts in the detail of what really could be captured by these optical elements. Using a technology called adaptive optics which is based on systems of deformable or mobile mirrors, astrophysical scientists attain to correct the distorted images of celestial bodies and determine the details of any form however diffuse it looks[1,2] **(Figs 1 and 2)**.

Joseff Bille, PhD, professor and physicist at the University of Heidelberg in Germany, is considered by many as the 'father' of wavefront technology applied to the research in the visual sciences. In this moment Dr Bille currently serves as the Director of the Institute of Applied Physics at the University of Heidelberg. In 1982 he registered the first

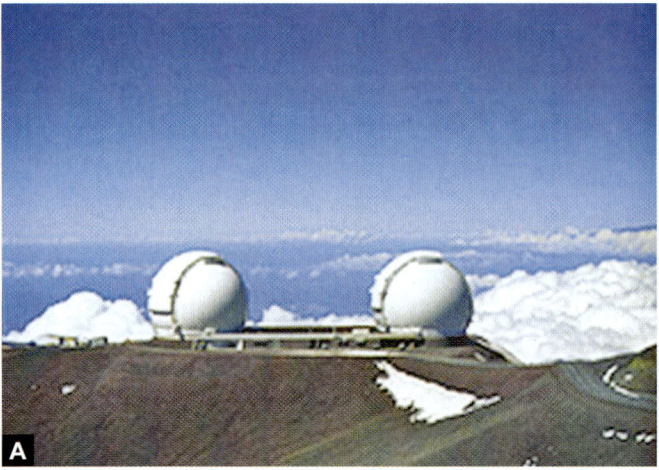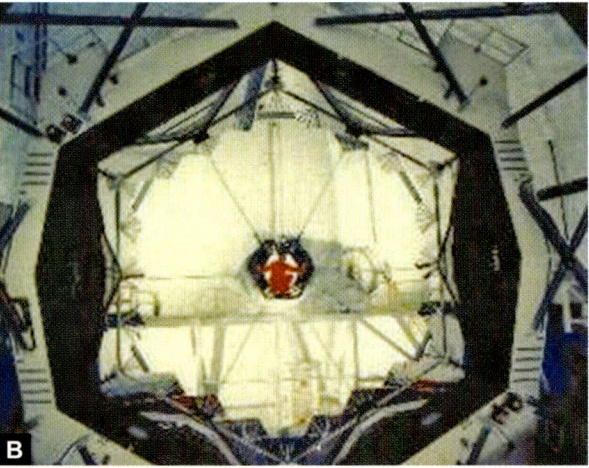

Figs 1A and B: (A) Keck I and II telescopes located on Mauna Kea (Hawaii); (B) Panel of hexagonal mirrors comprising the adaptive optics system compared to the size of a person (center of the figure)

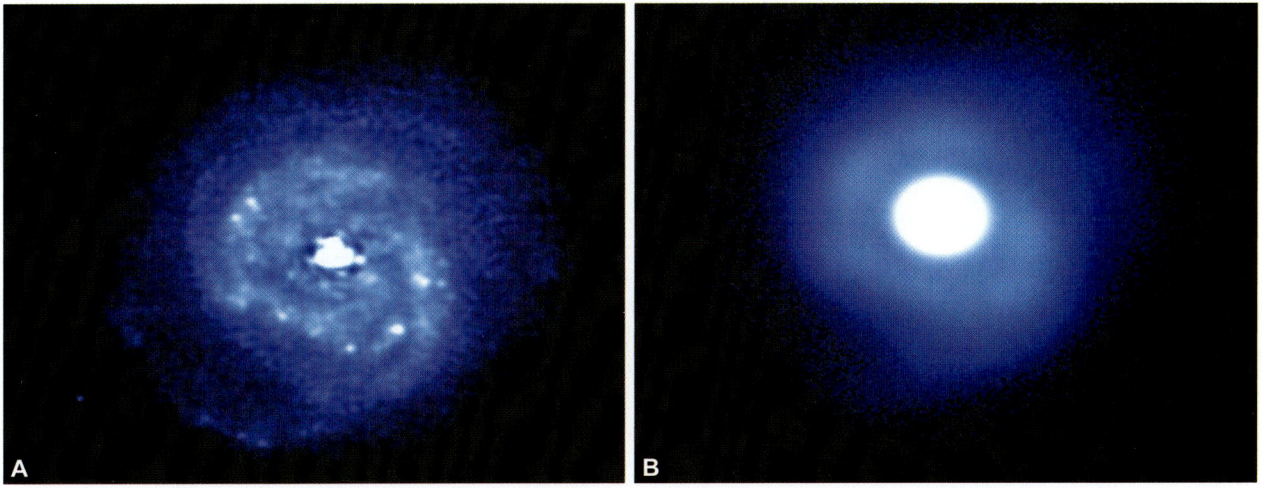

Figs 2A and B: Image of NGC 7469 galaxy view with and without adaptive optics

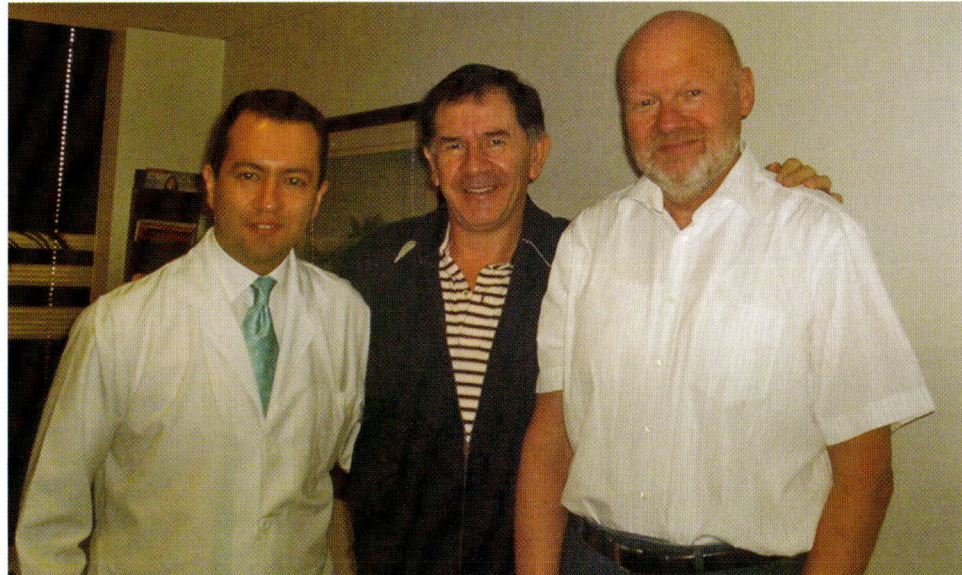

Fig. 3: From left to right: The author, Luis Antonio Ruiz MD, PhD and Professor Bille Joseff

patent about the applications of this technology in the field of visual sciences which was granted in 1986 by the German government. In 1997 becomes one of the cofounders of the 20/10 Club of Perfect Vision[1-3] **(Fig. 3)**.

It is important here to analyze what is the basic principle of the application of wavefront in the ocular optical system. Worth expressing in advance that there is no ideal optical system, but for purposes of study consider a perfect artificial eye such as the 'Indiana Eye' which is a mathematical scheme free from any kind of optical aberration and can be considered that its only optical limitation is the diffraction generated at the expense of the edge of the diaphragm (pupil). When in this perfect eye, parallel beams of object-image coming from the optical infinity refract, we can see that they all reach a same

focusing internal place that would be the equivalent to the macula in a biological eye, and if we could somehow analyze this output wavefront of the same optical system we would realize that this wavefront has not suffered any distortion and therefore the output beams are also parallel in the same way as they entered without undergoing any change.[3,4]

When analyzing an optical system in which aberrations exist, as could be an eye with some type of refractive error, irregularity or lack of transparent refractive media, we find that the light beams outgoing lose their parallelism and some of them are advanced with respect to the reference plane or delayed with respect to there. This is which we call deformity in wavefront or, etymologically, optical aberration **(Figs 4A and B)**.

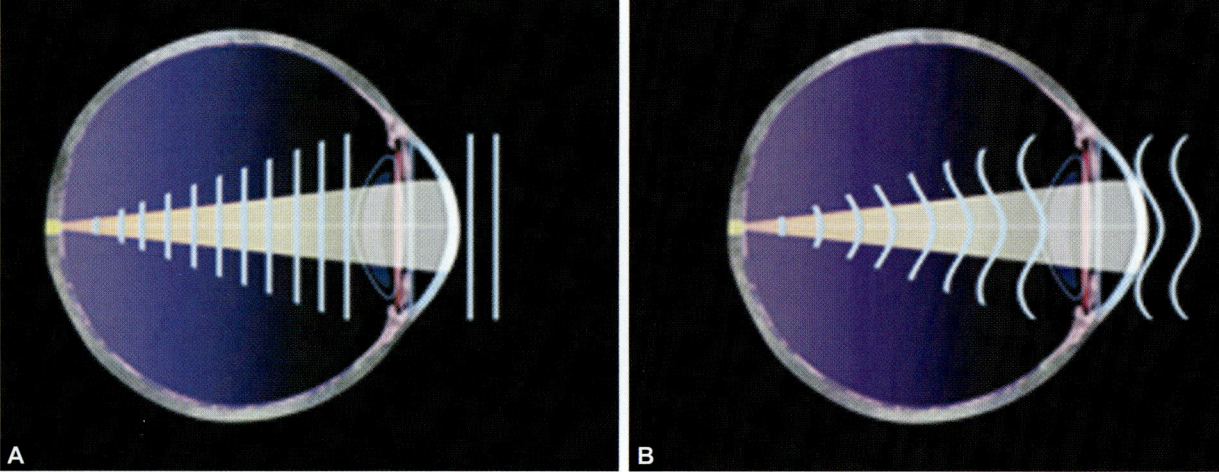

Figs 4A and B: (A) Perfect eye without aberrations; (B) Eye with aberrated wavefront

Each component of the optical system (optical train) pays a percentage of the wavefront distortion and this percentage depends directly on the relationship between the refracting surfaces (tear film, cornea, aqueous humor, lens and vitreous humor) and its refractive index.

From this point of view we can say that the tear film and the cornea are the refracting elements where the impact of the optical aberrations affects more on visual quality.

The tear film is where the biggest refractive index change occurs of all the optical train: from an index 1 corresponding to air to 1,336 corresponding to the corneal stroma, so the tear film has a key role and also dichotomous over the impact on visual quality: normal tear film has a constant thickness and has no optical effect in the perception of images and a tear film incomplete or poor in quality (dry eye) degrades the perceived image quality, because in this first interface, as said, occurs the highest index change of all refractive optical train.

Being the cornea a powerful refractive element (2/3 parts of total optical power of the eye) also is governed by a mathematical ratio regarding its contribution to the wavefront deformation: this ratio was described by Dr. Allain Telandro in Cannes (France) as 'the ratio 3 to 1' in which Dr. Telandro concludes that 3 microns of distortion in cornea generates 1 micron distortion in the wavefront.[3-5]

These deformities in the wavefront can be as complex as aberrated is the system that owns them. Depending on what the optical problem is based, certain types of alterations (aberrations) prevail on others, so that it is more or less deductible the aberration type to be found depending on the case being analyzed, by example myopic LASIK (positive spherical aberration), hyperopic LASIK (negative spherical aberration), keratoconus (coma and trefoil), dry eye (other of high order combined).[4-6]

ZERNIKE POLYNOMIALS

The Optical Society of America (OSA) recommended in the early interpreting wave front maps to adopt the expansion of Zernike polynomials as the standard method to describe the error in the wavefront of an optical system. Zernike polynomials are considered as the basic blocks of description or construction of any wavefront how complex it may be. Are known as *optical basic functions.*

Each of these basic functions is the product of other two functions, one of which depends only on the radio and the other on the meridian, this gives to the polynomials the mutual orthogonality characteristic, which means some are independent of other mathematically.

Another desirable feature of these polynomials is that, except for the first term, all have a zero mean and are scaled to have a variance corresponding to the unit. This puts all the terms in a common basis so that their relative magnitudes can be compared easily.[7-9]

The basic functions of Zernike or 'polynomials' as is often know are systematically arranged in a 'periodic table' with the shape of a pyramid.

Each row of the pyramid corresponds to a given order of the polynomial component of the function and each column corresponds to a different meridional frequency, by convention, the harmonics in cosine phase corresponds to positive frequencies and those in sine phase to negative frequencies. There is also a simpler way of placing each of these polynomial functions inside the pyramid and is giving it a simple ordinal number or even a double name with subscript and superscript indicating the exact position within the pyramid[8-10] **(Fig. 5).**

It is important to know that depending on the position of the aberration within the pyramid, this tends to deteriorate

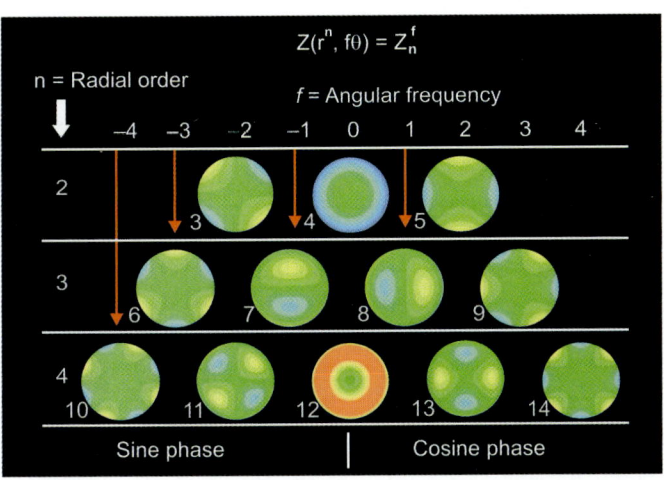

Fig. 5: Organization of Zernike polynomials in the pyramid

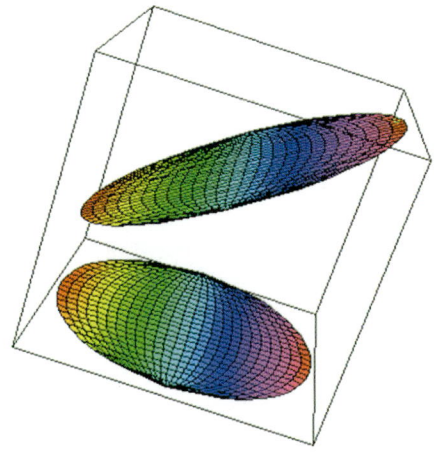

Fig. 6: Constant aberration tilt type

more or less the quality of the analyzed image. Thus it is considered that the more above the pyramid is placed an aberration and more centrally is located to the axis thereof, will have greater impact on the quality of patient's vision. As an example we then say that a pentafoil (peripheral aberration) of the same quantitative micron magnitude than a comma (central aberration) never distort the same way the quality of the vision of the analyzed system.

The wave front resulting in the quantitative analysis of the visual quality of a patient is the result of the mathematical sum of each of the polynomial expressions of Zernike pyramid, i.e. constant aberrations (Piston and Tilt), low-order aberrations (sphere and cylinder) and high-order aberrations (spherical aberration, coma, trefoil and other high-order ones).

The pyramid of polynomials then provides six different orders starting with zero order and can be considered divided into three main groups: constant aberrations, low-order aberrations and high-order ones.[7-10]

CONSTANT ABERRATIONS

Orders zero and one of the pyramid contain 3 aberrations that are considered constant in all optical systems and these are: the piston, horizontal tilt (Tilt) and the vertical tilt (Tip). The first one, the piston can be considered in its simplest form as the movement of internal focal plane in the attempt of the aberrometer optical system to conjugate with the retinal plane to capture the perceived image. The horizontal and vertical tilt aberrations are also constant, if we consider that our complex optical system is a symmetrically asymmetric system as the pupil has a certain asymmetry and is not in the mathematical center of the eye, like asymmetry characteristics of the cornea, of the lens, and the difference of the visual axis with the anatomical axis of the structures.

Considering these aberrations as constants in all optical systems we not generally take into account the total calculation of the aberrometry since its magnitude is so high that if you take it into account within the aberrometric calculation it would overshadow the detail and extent of the other distortions[7-10] **(Fig. 6)**.

LOW ORDER ABERRATIONS

Also known as second-order aberrations are the aberrations we know in our diagnostic and therapeutic reality daily.

They are three expressions that occupy this second order: two components of astigmatism and a spherical blur component or defocus. These are the aberrations that we are used to measure, correct and deal with glasses, contact lenses or conventional refractive surgery.

It is important to understand at this point that low-order aberrations aberrometrically represent the amount of vision or quantification of the sphero cylindrical defect.

Astigmatism has two expressions used to determine its magnitude and its axis as follows: from the sum of the first term and the second, we obtain the magnitude of astigmatism as we know it and of the percentage respect to one another is determined its axis. Regarding defocus or spherical blur we mention that aberrometrically represents the error of the central rays of a wave front respect to the peripherals and this in turn can be positive or negative (if this is a myopic or hyperopic error).

To better understand the dimensions of a low-aberration order is necessary to note that these aberrometrical maps are built based on advanced or delayed microns with respect to a zero reference plane. By convention as a similar way to construct corneal elevation maps, the representation of the referential aberrometrical plane is given by variations in color tone, in the green range is shown a zero level of measure in microns, the 'hot' colors in the range of yellows, oranges and reds with their various tones representing the wave front advancing in microns or that is considered faster with respect to the zero reference plane, and in turn 'cool' colors show the slow or delayed wave front in microns respect to the ideal plane.

SECTION 2

In this way, if we represent bidimensionally an aberrometrical map of astigmatism this would have the shape of a curved plane alternately towards and forth. Its three-dimensional representation would be a figure described by some as the 'saddle' where a fast front alternates with a slow one **(Figs 7A to C)**.

The two-dimensional representation of a myopic spherical defect would show a wavefront fast in the periphery, that is progressively slowing as it approaches the center of the optical axis of the system. The three-dimensional representation of this front will display a figure that has been described as a 'bowl' shape. The reason for this is that in the myopic patient, rays that go through the axial center of the system must go a distance much longer than the rays of the periphery and therefore these leave long before the eye and reach prior the aberrometer sensor than those that are located in the central part of the pupil. Similar but opposite is the case of hyperopia in which we can consider its three-dimensional wavefront as a 'bowl' but seen by the base, in which we have a fast wavefront at the center to be progressively slowing towards the periphery[7-10] **(Figs 7A to C)**.

HIGHER-ORDER ABERRATIONS

From the third order we find a number that is progressively expanding the length of the pyramid and in fact this expansion may become infinite, but for practical purposes of the human optical analysis is only considered important to the sixth order and even some researchers claim that the analysis of the expressions only to the fourth order is sufficient when it comes to optical measurements of visual quality. The sum of the high-order aberrations quantifies irregular astigmatism in an optical system, which is directly related to the objective visual quality.

Irregular astigmatism or so-called High Order aberrations are the Visual Function part that we are not used to measure or to treat and that now with wavefront technology and customized ablations we try to measure and correct for carrying to not previously thought limits the vision quality of our patients, as well as understanding new concepts of our limited knowledge of the objective visual quality. It is considered that in a normal eye, low-order aberrations constitute 80–85 percent of deteriorating Visual Quantity and that high-order aberrations constitute only 15% of the total error (Visual Quality).[9,10]

Despite the significant difference in these variables percentage these high-order aberrations are those that limit the vision of a healthy eye below the retinal limit and can be said that they are not susceptible to correct with conventional methods.[11]

Trefoil is the first of these aberrations, also known by some as triangular astigmatism, represents bidimensionally the alternation forward-backward of three fixed points which define a steepening of the plane at the expense of the periphery. Its three-dimensional image represents an advancing wave front that delays and alternate on 3 occasions at the expense of periphery **(Figs 8A and B)**.

The Coma is considered perhaps one of the most fearsome aberrations within the spectrum of high-order aberrations due to the significant visual quality deterioration that its finding represents, when induced by a surgical or therapeutic procedure. Moderate natural coma however, seems to be related with good visual acuities as in the case of emmetropic airline pilots with excellent visual acuity in which is found that this was the most frequent aberration **(Figs 8A and B).**

Throughout his speech the comma represents the offset of the elements constituting an optical system, hence its importance as contributing to the deterioration of visual quality. This aberration is an important finding in patients with diseases such as asymmetric keratoconus, where becomes a sensitive marker of its presence. Or in patients with offset refractive treatments or inclined intraocular lenses or out of position.[14-16]

Bidimensionally coma displays from the periphery to the center a split wavefront alternating horizontally or vertically (depending on the type of coma), in planes that move or are

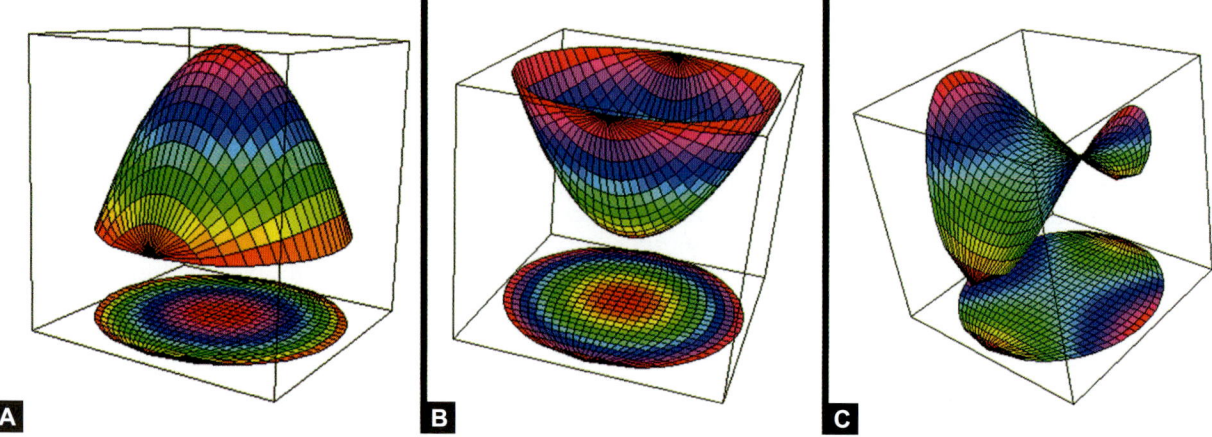

Figs 7A to C: Low order aberrations: three-dimensional representation of hyperopic, myopic and astigmatic defect

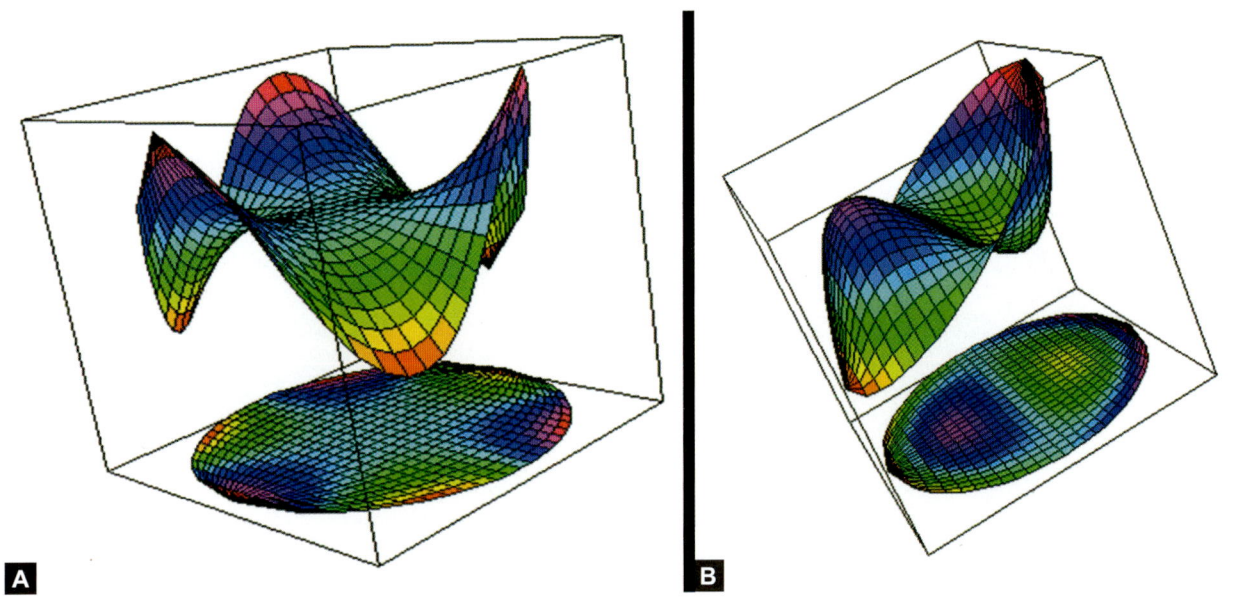

Figs 8A and B: High order aberrations: (A) Trefoil; (B) Coma

delayed abruptly. In a three-dimensional representation, this wave front reveals a sharp breaking with deep undulations alternating forward—backward from the center to the periphery.

The Tetrafoil or quadratic astigmatism, is located in the fourth order and has two expressions for the angular frequency of sine and cosine respectively, in a similar way and progressive as trefoil, is the peripheral aberration that represents the symmetry of four fixed points at the expense of periphery and in its two and three dimensional form represents a wave front advancing and is delayed in four opportunities on the periphery of the analyzed area **(Figs 9A and B)**.

Spherical aberration is located inside the pyramid in the fourth radial order with angular frequency zero. Spherical aberration is a symmetric aberration and is defined as the focal distance between the center points and the periphery of a wave front, if the center and periphery of a system become more curved, spherical aberration becomes greater.

The human eye handles positive spherical aberration naturally and has different elements that are optically evolved to control or minimize the impact of this aberration in visual quality, in fact mechanisms to be mentioned reduce to one third the amount of spherical aberration of an optical system when doing analysis in a young healthy eye. An important mechanism of control is the 'Aspheric' shape in the cornea, the flattening of the radius of curvature of the cornea from the center towards the periphery, enables both beams, central and peripheral to occupy the same position in the macular focal plane improving the quantity of useful light (irradiance) for the formation of the image.

The other mechanism of spherical aberration compensation comes at the expense of the lens by virtue of the curvature of its front and back face as well as the refractive index difference between the central area and periphery.[4,11,12]

Aberrometrically the bidimensional analysis of this type of optical distortion shows an image with cool colors on the periphery of wavefront which increases gradually towards the center, its three-dimensional classical shape describes it as a 'Mexican hat'.

It is important to know that this aberration as others described above are related directly to their quantitative impact on visual quality factors depending on the size of the pupil, so large pupils contribute with a higher percentage of aberrations in optical systems than systems with small pupils.[18-21]

Typically is described that conventional techniques of LASIK can increase the presence of this kind of aberration due to micro offsets of treatments or due to the size of the optical zone[22] **(Figs 9A and B)**.

Insofar as we descend progressively in the analysis of the aberrations in the pyramid, each of these aberrations presents its secondary component, which is a variation in shape of the primary. Also can be located in sine or cosine phase (except for the zero symmetry aberrations—center of the pyramid) and be negative or positive. This would give for each of the majority of aberrations 4 possible terms with which could be described its position, nature and symmetry through combinations thereof.[13] For example:

Zero symmetry aberration: Primary spherical aberration, secondary spherical aberration, positive spherical aberration, negative spherical aberration.

Asymmetric aberrations: Primary coma, secondary coma, coma in sine phase coma in cosine phase.

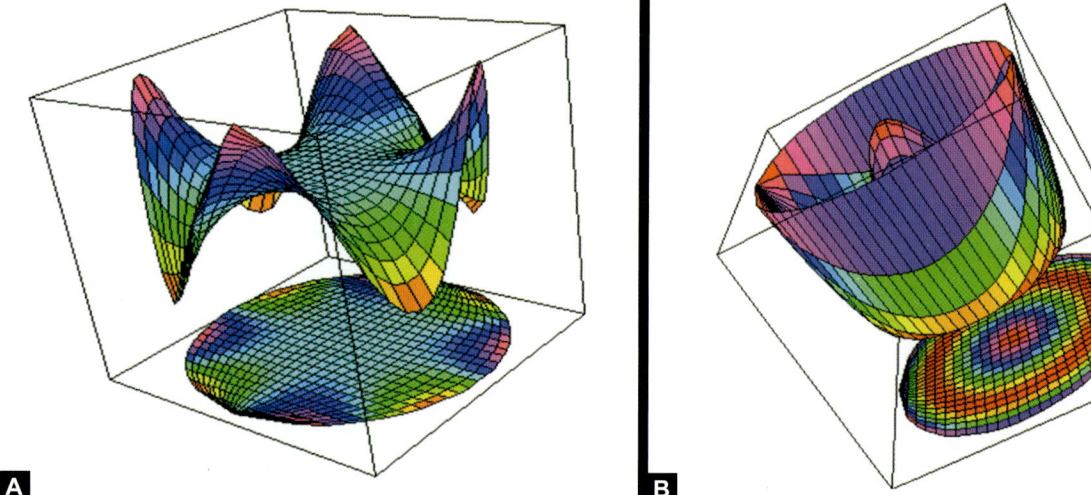

Figs 9A and B: High order aberrations: (A) Tetrafoil; (B) Spherical aberration

OBJECTIVE VISUAL QUALITY MEASURES

Although this type of objective measure of visual quality through aberrometric tests provides different numerical data as information, we will make special mention of some terms considered important and representative of a wavefront analysis.[3,5,6,8]

The objective visual quality measures can be quantified numerically at pupil or retinal level.

Pupil Level

Pupil as a dynamic diaphragm that allows passage of light is considered of vital importance in quantifying the objective visual quality.

Pupils with sizes greater than 6 mm in diameter are considered large from the refractive and aberrometric point of view, this means that the optical systems that have these large pupils may be mostly subject to the impact of the objective visual quality deterioration in terms of maximum dilation (e.g. mesopic or scotopic condition in myopic), instead patients with small pupils less than 3 mm have a low impact on visual.

quality at the expense of the aberrations, but are subject to the limitation by the diffraction generated by the pupillary margin *per se*.

There is a pupil size of 'balance' between the limited size by aberrations and diffraction limited size and this is equal to 4 mm diameter.

An important condition for taking an aberrometric test is total absence of natural or artificial ambient light. This allows the examination to be made on the condition of maximum natural pupillary dilation, the aberrometric test result always expresses measurement results based on the higher obtained pupil under this minimal luminous condition, but it is also important to know that any aberrometer can recalculate the

wave front for a pupil diameter we arbitrary have chosen. This feature may be selected for example in visual quality studies (e.g. refractive surgery results, performance of intraocular lenses, etc.).

Root mean square—average square error (RMS): A term that could be considered complicated in its definition is just the average mathematical quantification of the error in the wavefront.

Represents the square sum of each of the polynomial terms in the Zernique pyramid being studied and the square root expression of this summation. Its value is absolute and it is considered that the RMS is the numerical representation of the amount of error of an ideal wave front respect to the patient studied. The RMS of an ideal optical system is zero, but as said earlier this ideal system does not exist.

The RMS is considered an objective quantitative measurement of visual quality at pupillary plane level.

The RMS can be analyzed from the context of sum of all aberrations of a system and is called total RMS or from the point of analysis of single high-order aberrations where RMS is described as RMSHO (higher order or irregular astigmatism RMS).

The total RMS of a human emmetropic optical system is considered equal to unity (1) measured in microns, if less than one can say that this eye sees beyond the one hundred percent and if it is greater than unity indicates a deterioration of the quality of patient's vision.

Total RMS	Visual acuity
1.5 microns	20/80
1.0 microns	20/20
0.5 microns	20/15

Moreover, the RMS can be analyzed individually or in subgroups depending on the detail of the clinical-optical analysis being performed.

The high-order RMS or RMS HO only quantifies high order aberrations, in other words, irregular astigmatism and therefore becomes an important objective measure of visual quality, multiple studies confirm that in normal populations the cutoff of this type RMS is 0.4 microns, this means that patients with RMS HO with values below 0.4 microns can be considered with a normal or low irregular astigmatism and therefore with a normal or high visual quality. Whereas patients with RMS HO greater than 0.4 microns may have some alteration of optical components which impairs the visual quality. These patients should undergo careful clinical analysis to determine the cause of impairment in the objective visual quality.[11,13]

I had just spoken of the "single qualitative weight" of each aberration: and we can say that even when two individual aberrations have the same numerical magnitude of RMS in microns, they will not have the same impact on the visual quality of the individual.

The individual RMS of each aberration separately is considered maximum to 0.18 microns, this means that in the individual analysis of each aberration. In polynomials Zernique pyramid, there should not be a value greater than this for every single term, for example, spherical aberration greater than 0.18 microns could be related to a prior refractive procedure, vertical coma greater than 0.18 micras could be related to the early presence of keratoconus.[11]

Retinal Level

Point Spread Function (PSF)

The spread function of a point, is an objective measure of the visual quality quantification at retinal plane level. Considering the PSF as the measure of the dispersion of an object-image with the shape of a point at the plane of focus on the retina. Optical system without aberrations is able to perceive a luminous point as a point, while an aberrated optical system induce significant changes in the perception of this point.

A suitable PSF should consider features such as its high contrast and compact form. The compact form (volume) is directly related with the quality of the image that is forming in the retina of the optical system examined: the more compact the better the quality of the vision of this system. The high contrast defines the amount of light energy (irradiance) that is transmitted to the retina or macular attachment point **(Fig. 10)**

Optical Transfer Function (OTF)

The efficiency of transfer of images through an optical system should be evaluated in two ways: the transfer process itself

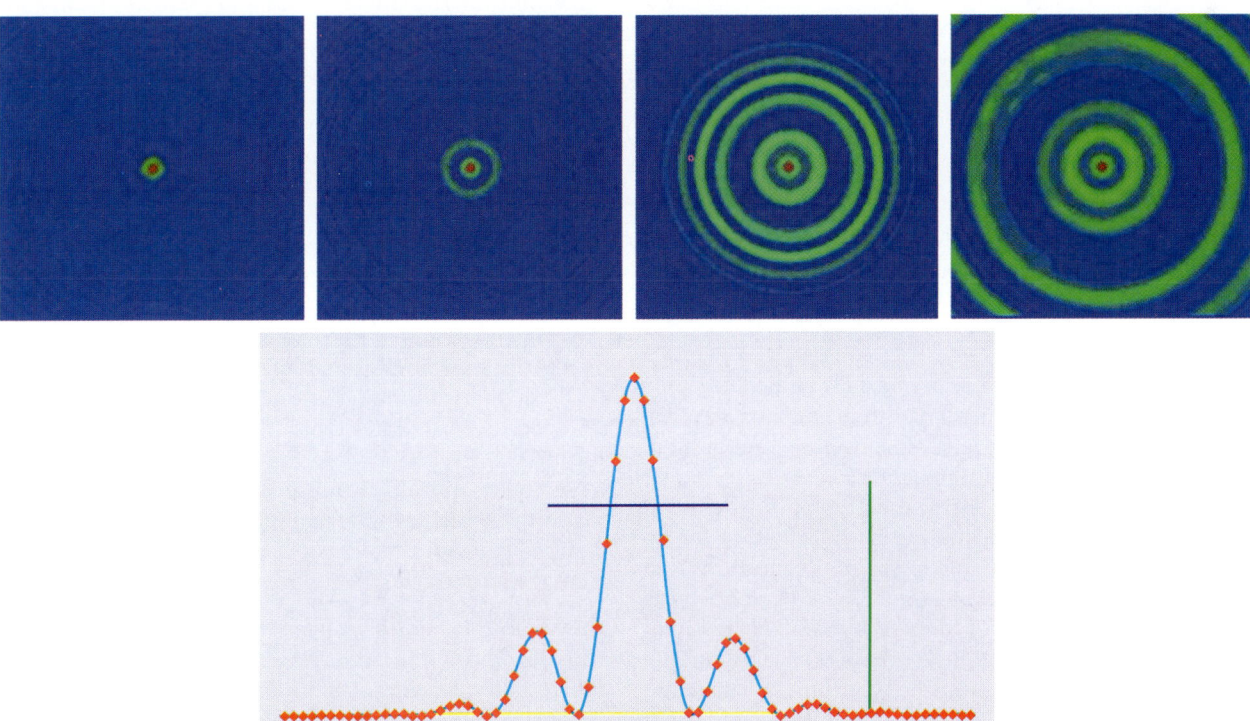

Fig. 10: Point spread function horizontal line—volume and vertical line: irradiance or energy that reaches the retina

and the quality of images transferred through the system in question. This is accomplished by analyzing the ability to transfer different images with sinusoidal characteristics and with different spatial frequencies.

Phase Transfer Function (PTF)

Represents a simple lateral displacement of a sinusoidal image of specific spatial frequency, observed through an aberrated system.

Modulated Transfer Function (MTF)

It is defined as the quantified ability to transfer a specific image through an optical system with a specific resolution and contrast. In other words the amount of image transmitted from the observed object through an aberrated optical system (refracting elements of the eye) to the photoreceptor (retina).

Aberrometry Limitations

As far wavefront measurement is a science of new application in our ophthalmologic field, is important to know the reality of the historic moment we are living with this brand new technology and though this development promises offer significant advances in terms of study and understanding of the role of visual quality and also personalized treatments with refractive surgery, it is considered that this is a science developing in their ocular applications and therefore should be at aware of the limitations that wavefront measures can have at some point.[22-25]

Tear Film

The tear film is considered the first refracting surface of eye with all known importance because it is the area which holds the most drastic change in terms of refractive indices (refractive index of air = 1, refractive index of the tear film = 1.336).

It is well-known by everyone in our daily clinical practice the important subjective annoyance that patients manifest with some degree of dry eye and constant complaint of fluctuating vision or loss of visual quality.[17]

In this same way, a wavefront measure in an eye with poor tear film can dramatically affect the outcome of an aberrometry and induce multiple high-order distortions that should constitute an irregular astigmatism induced by micro differences in the thickness of the tear film and consequent loss of the homogeneity of the surface of corneal epithelium.

Considering the quality of the tear film as a major constraint of aberrometrical measurement is also true that the aberrometers with which the market has are sensitive enough to monitor and quantify optical changes associated with the disruption of the tear.

This so, an important limitation of the aberrometry can be converted in the future in a valuable technique to understand changes in visual quality related to dry eye **(Fig. 11)**.

Pupil Size

The contour or an aberrometric map and the aberrations there found can change significantly depending on with pupil size measurement is made, since a small change in millimeters of pupillar diameter may represent huge variations in terms of square area of its circular shape. Also worth bearing in mind the diffractive effect that the edge of the pupil exerts on light beams that constitute the aberrometer measurement and limit the quality of the aberrometrical acquisition in very small pupils or distort data in very large pupils or pharmacologically dilated. That is why perhaps most aberrometrical systems manufacturers, with the exception of a few, suggests that an ideal aberroscopic measurement should be made in scotopic conditions without action of drugs that dilate the pupil **(Figs 12A and B)**.

Chromatic Aberration

Aberrometric technology with which we currently use, mostly uses coherent and monochromatic wavelengths based on the principle and application of laser wavelengths, typically in the infrared range.

These laser beams to measure the distortion of the wavefront have a single wavelength, which is constant and does not change in its entry or exit path. It is important to note here that the many wavelengths of a multicolor world occupy different focusing places in the thickness of the retina, so the lengths of short wavelengths in the blue spectrum are focused on the anterior part of the retina, the medium wavelength in the yellow and orange spectrum focus on the middle part of the retina and finally long wavelengths corresponding to the range of colors in the red spectrum focus more on the retina after. Aberrations and RMS tend to increase to the extent that the wavelength also increases.

Unfortunately not exist at the time an aberrometer to be able to measure all the spectrum of visible light and its single drive in a human optic system. Aberrometers spatially resolved, experimental type, after complex measures have succeeded in giving information to 6 various different wavelengths, but this is not possible with technology that is currently available in the market.

Aberrometer Sensors Resolution

This is an inherent characteristic of construction, principle and density of the sensors with which is constituted the aberrometer, it is important to know that the greater number of sensors better the measuring at the expense of one more detailed description of what the wavefront can be and the specific quantification of each Zernike polynomials that constituent.

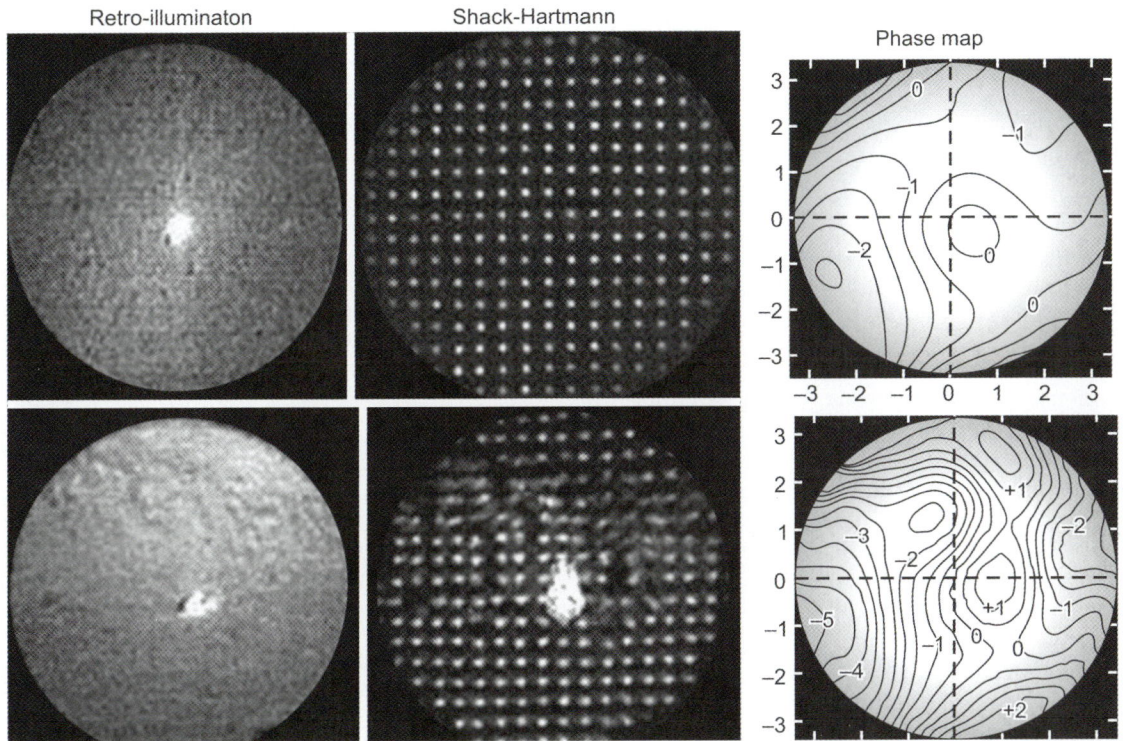

Fig. 11: Images: backlight centroids of Shack-Hartmann system and map of densities in the same patient after 40 seconds without blinking

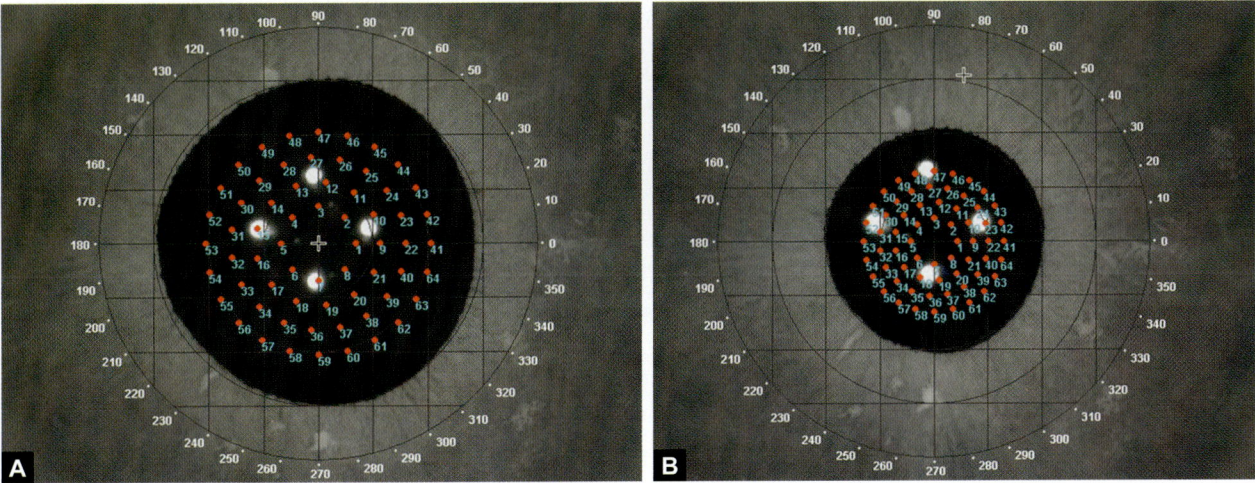

Figs 12A and B: Aberrometric test results with different pupil size

The aberrometric measurement principles can be classified for practical purposes from the point of view of the place where the machine captures the image to be analyzed, according to this are called: of internal process (ingoing process) or of external process (outgoing process); in the first group of aberrometers image capturing is done at the retinal plane and in the second at the output level of the pupil. In a separate group we found the schiascopic aberrometers, the spatially resolved (experimental) and for aberrometric calculation from high-resolution corneal topography.[24-32]

- **Internal process (ingoing process)**
  - Tscherning
  - Ray tracing
- **External process (outgoing process)**
  - Hartman-Shack
- **Schiascopic**
  - Dynamic retinoscopy

SECTION 2

- **Spatially resolved:** It is considered the only subjective aberrometer, experimental use
- **Corneal aberrometers:** Based on high-resolution corneal topography (not real aberrometers)

The density of the number of sensors also speaks of the richness of the information with which to build aberrometrical data. One way to express is as from the measure of the aberrometer resolution, which is expressed in microns and tells us that with a fewer resolution in microns image quality measured is better.

CONCLUSION

The aberrometry, new diagnostic trend, heritage of astrophysics, has aroused curiosity and loathing in ophthalmology colleagues, many of them interested in this new science as another way to analyze the visual function, others are not at all interested for the difficult terminology of their slang or by complex mathematical concepts underlying. With the advent of multiple aberrometric systems in the diagnosis and therapeutic arsenal in refractive surgery, it is important to know in detail the principle and the foundations of this new branch of knowledge of visual quality. We believe that venture into this new world with solid basic knowledge and easily explained, help to understand more easily a fascinating universe of optical functions.

REFERENCES

1. Howard C Howland. The history and methods of ophthalmic wavefront sensing. J Refract Surg. 2000;16:S552-3.
2. Aberraciones que es eso de lo que habla todo el mundo?: Manual Básico de Supervivencia., Pablo Artal, Comunicado Ver y Oír, Marzo de 2002.
3. Benjamin F Boyd. Wavefront Analysis: Aberrómetros y Topografía Corneal. Highlights of Ophthalmology International, Primera edicion en español, 2003.
4. Antonio Calossi. Corneal asphericity and spherical aberration. J Refract Surg. 2007;23:505-14.
5. Susana Marcos, Stephen A Burns, Esther Moreno-Barriusop, Rafael Navarro. A new approach to the study of ocular chromatic aberrations. Vision Research. 1999; 39:4309-23.
6. Heidi Hofer, Pablo Artal, Ben Singer, Juan Luis Aragón, David R. Williams. Dynamics of the eye's wave aberration. J Opt Soc Am. 2001;18(3):497-506.
7. Larry N Thibos, Raymond A Applegate, James T Schwiegerling, Robert Webb. Report from the VSIA taskforce on standards for reporting optical aberrations of the eye. J Refract Surg. 2000;16:S654-5.
8. Guang-ming Dai. Comparison of wavefront reconstructions with zernike polynomials and fourier transforms. J Refract Surg. 2006;22:943-8.
9. Larry N Thibos, Raymond A Applegate, James T Schwiegerling, Robert Webb. Standards for reporting the optical aberrations of eyes. J Refract Surg. 2002;18:S652-60.
10. Larry N Thibos. Wavefront Data Reporting and Terminology. J Refract Surg. 2001;17:S578-83.
11. Raymond A Applegate, Edwin J Sarver, Vic Khemsara. Are all aberrations equal? J Refract Surg. 2002;18:S556-62.
12. Marine Gobbe, Michel Guillon, Cecile Maissa. Measurement repeatability of corneal aberrations. J Refract Surg. 2002;18: S567-71.
13. Andrew B Watson, Albert J Ahumada. Predicting visual acuity from wavefront aberrations. J of Vision. 2008;8(4);17:1-19.
14. Jorge L Alió, Mohamed H Shabayek. Corneal higher order aberrations a method to grade keratoconus. J Refract Surg. 2006;22:539-45.
15. Batool Jafri, Xiaohui Li, Huiying Yang, Yaron S Rabinowitz. Higher order wavefront aberrations and topography in early and suspected keratoconus. J Refract Surg. 2007;23:774-81.
16. Ramkumar Sabesan. Visual performance after correcting HOAs in keratoconic eyes. J of Vision. 2009;9(5);6:1-10.
17. Lung-Kun Yeh, Cheng-Jen Chiu, Chieh-Fang Fong, I-Jong Wang, Wei-Li Chen, Chuhsing Kate Hsiao, Samuel CM Huang, Yung-Feng Shih, Fung-Rong Hu, Luke LK Lin. The genetic effect on refractive error and anterior corneal aberration twin eye study. J Refract Surg. 2007;23:257-65.
18. Sabong Srivannaboon, Dan Z Reinstein, Timothy J Archer. Diurnal variation of higher order aberrations in human eyes. J Refract Surg. 2007;23:442-6.
19. Ioannis G Pallikaris, Sophia I Panagopoulou, Charalambos S Siganos, Vasilys V Molebny. Objective measurement of wavefront aberrations with and without accommodation. J Refract Surg. 2001;17:S602-7.
20. Hang Cheng, Raymond Applegate. A population study on changes in wave aberrations with accommodation. J of Vision. 2004;4:272-80.
21. Krisztina Hagyó, Béla Csákány, Zsolt Lang, János Németh. Variability of higher order wavefront aberrations after blinks. J Refract Surg. 2009;25:59-68.
22. Susana Marcos. Aberrations and visual performance following standard laser vision correction. J Refract Surg. 2001;17:S596-S601.
23. Alejandro Cerviño, Sarah L Hosking, Robert Montes-Mico, Keith Bates. Clinical ocular wavefront analyzers. J Refract Surg. 2007;23:603-16.
24. Michael Mrochen. Revealing company secrets—please tell the truth and nothing but the truth! J Refract Surg. 2000;16:S654-9.
25. Pablo Rodríguez, Rafael Navarro, Justo Arines, Salvador Bará. A new calibration set of phase plates for ocular aberrometers. J Refract Surg. 2006;22:275-84.
26. Stephen A Burns. The spatially resolved refractometer. J Refract Surg. 2000;16:S566-9.
27. Michael Mrochen, Maik Kaemmerer, Peter Mierdel, Hans-Eberhard Krinke, Theo Seiler. Principles of Tscherning aberrometry. J Refract Surg. 2000;16:S570-1.
28. Vasyl V Molebny, Sophia I Panagopoulou, Sergiy V Molebny, Youssef S Wakil, Ioannis G Pallikaris. Principles of ray tracing aberrometry. J Refract Surg. 2000;16:S572-5.
29. Paul D Pulaski, James T Roller, Daniel R Neal, Keith Ratte. Measurement of aberrations with microlenses using a Shack-Hartmann wavefront sensor. J Optal Soc America. 1980;70(8).
30. Larry N Thibos. Principles of Hartmann-Shack aberrometry. J Refract Surg. 2000;16:S565-3.
31. Ahmet Z Burakgazi, Bernard Tinio, Alejandro Bababyan, Kevin Kevork Niksarli, Penny Asbell. Higher order aberrations in normal eyes measured with three different aberrometers. J Refract Surg. 2006;22:898-903.
32. Alejandro Cervino, Sarah L Hosking, Gurjeet K Rai, Shezhad A Naroo, Bernard Gilmartin. Wavefront analyzers induce instrument myopia. J Refract Surg. 2006;22:795-803.

CHAPTER 6

Wavefront Aberrations from A to Z

Yazan A Zahran

INTRODUCTION

Before we start talking about wavefront we should mention that to understand wavefront aberrations, we should change our thinking about light, light is expressed differently in geometrical and physical optics. The rays from a point source of light radiates out in all directions in geometrical optics. In physical optics, conversely light is considered as a wave and the light wave spreads in all directions as a spherical wave. The wavefront is the shape of the light waves that are all in-phase. Although light coming from infinity is considered to be linear bundles of light rays. It also expressed as a plane wavefront (wavefront is a continuous surface that propagates perpendicular to the direction of the lights rays) **(Fig. 1)**.

FACTORS AFFECT THE OPTICAL QUALITY OF THE RETINAL IMAGE

- Diffraction
- Whole eye wavefront error (wavefront aberration) that will be discussed in this chapter
- Scatter
- Chromatic aberration.

Wavefront Basics

So the main question is what do we mean by wavefront aberrations? To define the concept of wavefront aberration, it is necessary to define the wavefront of a point light source, and before that the concepts of optical path length (OPL) and the optical path difference (OPD).

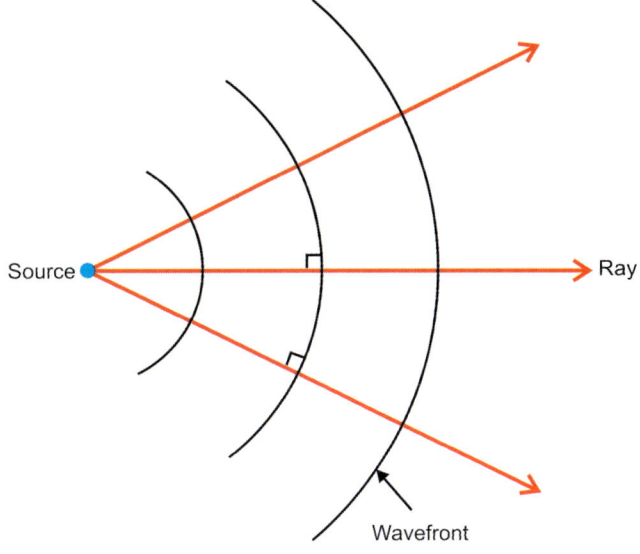

Fig. 1: Linear rays

From a clinical perspective, one of the most useful ways to interpret the wavefront aberration function is the differences in the optical path length (OPL) traveled by rays as they pass from object to image, OPL is a measurement of the number of oscillations of a light wave that propagates from point to another.

A propagating wavefront of light is defined by a collection of points in space that are found at the same OPL of a common light source to define the aberration of an optical system, the OPL of a ray that passes through any point (x, y) of the pupil plane can be compared to a main ray, which passes through the center of the pupil (0, 0) as this light ray is not deviated nor distorted along its path. The result is the OPD.

In a perfect optical system, the OPL will be the same for all light rays that travel from a point on an object to a point on the image, so the OPD is 0 for all positions (x, y) on the pupil. These rays will have the same phase and will therefore aggregate constructively to produce the perfect image for an eye focused on infinity, the ideal wavefront exiting from an aberration-free eye is flat and circular (**Fig. 2**).

On the other hand, light that passes through different points on the pupil will arrive at the destination in different phases. Consequently, the system is aberrated and the quality of the image will be distorted. So if we consider aberrations as being the difference in OPL it stands to reason that the aberrations could derive from the qualitative and quantitative anomalies of the lacrimal film, the cornea, the aqueous humor, the crystalline lens, the vitreous body, decentering or

inclination of the various optical components of the eye and each component's relationship to the others (**Fig. 3**).

So to sum up wavefront aberration is defined as the optical path difference (OPD) between the ideal and the actual (aberrated) wavefront (**Figs 4A and B**).

Classification of Aberrations

We can classify wavefront aberration into:
- Low order aberrations (0-2 radial order) include refractive defects that can be corrected with spectacles or standard contact lenses.
- High order aberrations (more than second radial order) include spherical aberrations, coma and all aberrations that are classed under the heading of irregular astigmatism or defects that cannot be corrected with commercially available spectacles or lenses.

We can classify the aberration further into monochromatic or polychromatic:
- Monochromatic aberrations are associated with a specific wavelength.
- Polychromatic aberrations is caused by the dispersion of light in various media it crosses and the light will spilt into various colors of the visible spectrum.

Fig. 2: The relationship between the wavefront and the light rays. The light rays travel perpendicular to the wavefront at all points

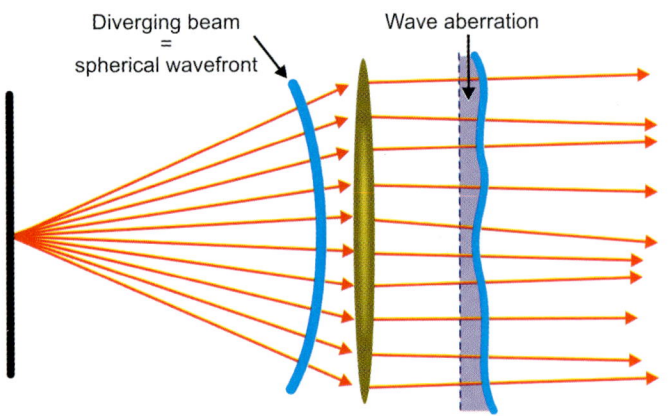

Fig. 3: The wavefront aberrations, illustrated in gray, is the difference between the ideal wavefront and aberrated wavefront

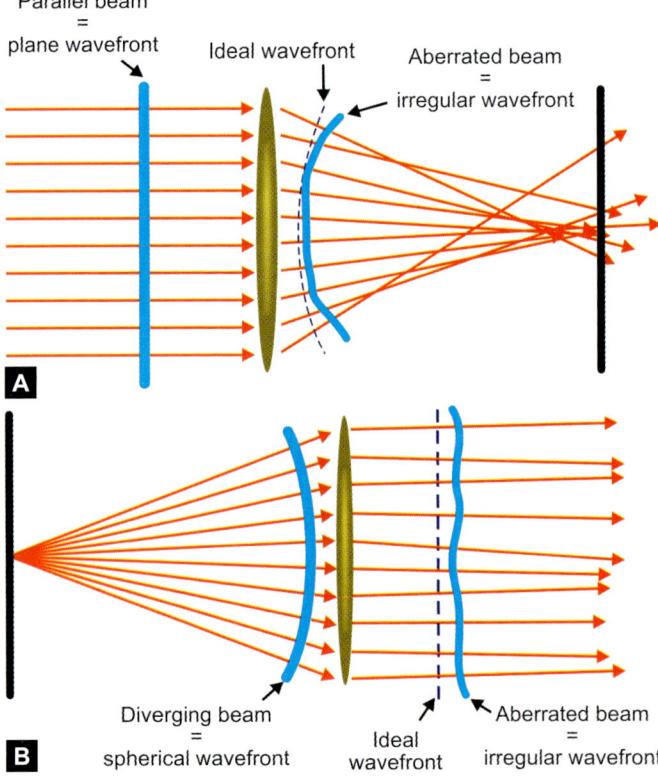

Figs 4A and B: The emerging light in these two images neither converges to a point nor does it form a parallel beam, resulting in irregular-shaped wavefront

We can classify aberrations according the site of origin of the aberrations which include:

- Corneal aberrations
- Internal optics aberrations
- Total ocular aberrations which include the sum of the corneal and the internal optics aberrations **(Fig. 5)**.

Representing Wavefront Aberrations

For wavefront measurement to be useful in the analysis of vision, aberration must be represented by terms that can be understood by ophthalmologist here comes the role of the Zernike and Fourier series polynomials and in simple words both Zernike and Fourier describe complex three-dimensional surfaces in mathematical terms, making it possible to design customized corneal ablation.

The Zernike polynomials are the most widely adopted tool to describe wavefront aberration, this mathematical method considers every map as the adjusted sum of fundamental shapes or the basic functions as shown in the figure below.

These group of mathematical expressions are the product of two functions-one of which depends solely on the R radius of a point on the pupil, and the other depends solely on the θ meridian of a point on the pupil plane. The first function is a simple polynomial of the nth degree and the second is the harmonic of a sinusoid or co-sinusoid.

The double index model Z(r, f) where the index r describes the higher power (order) of the radial polynomials and the index f described the Azimuthal frequency of the sinusoidal component. The basic Zernike functions or modes or terms are systematically grouped on a pyramid-shaped periodic table. Each line of the pyramid corresponds to a given order of the polynomial of the function and each column corresponds to the different Azimuthal frequency. By convention the harmonics in the cosine phase are identified with plus sign while those in the sine phase are identified with minus sign. The unit of measurement for every Zernike coefficient is the micron.

Polynomials can be expanded up to any arbitrary order if sufficient numbers of measurements for calculations are made.

Measurement of Wavefront Aberrations

Wavefront sensing techniques can be categorized by whether the measurement is based on subjective or objective methods. It is difficult to measure the wavefront aberrations accurately using subjective methods due to prolonged measurement period and its dependence on the subject's judgment.

Wavefront sensors usually use ray-tracing methods to reconstruct the wavefront and are classified into the following three types:

1. Outgoing wavefront aberrometry is used in the Hartmann-Shack sensor.
2. Ingoing retinal imaging aberrometry is used in the cross cylinder aberroscope, the Tscherning aberroscope and the sequential ray tracing method.
3. The ingoing feedback aberrometer is used in the spatially resolved refractometer (SRR). The optical path difference method (OPD) (slit retinoscopy or skiascopy) is a variant of this method.

6

CHAPTER

Wavefront components

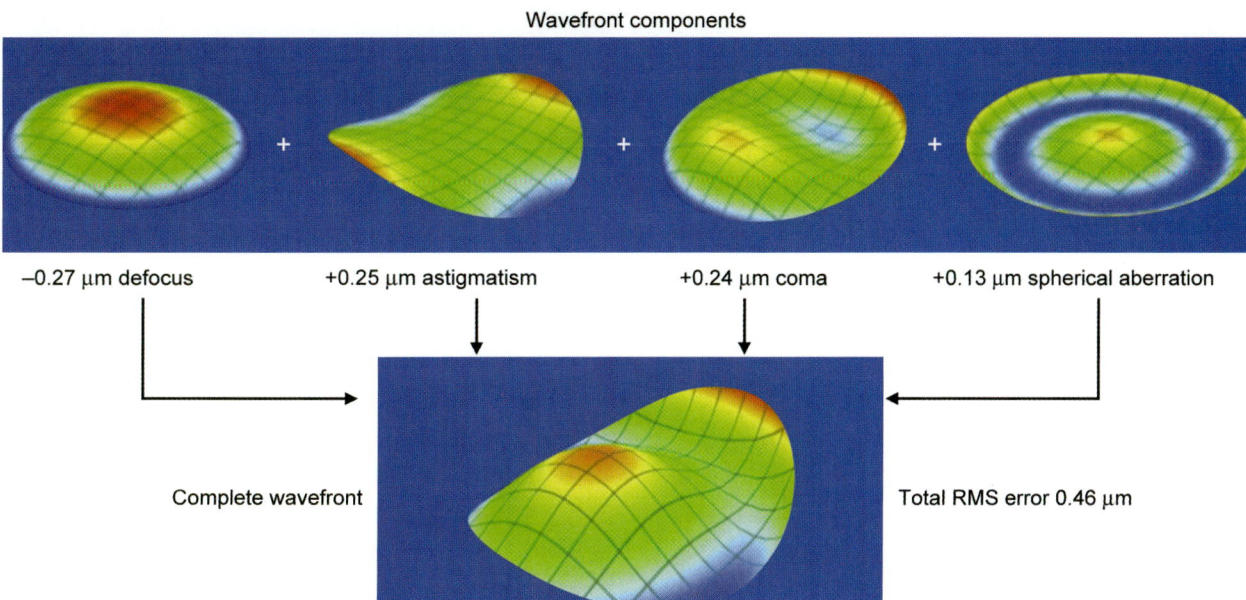

−0.27 µm defocus   +0.25 µm astigmatism   +0.24 µm coma   +0.13 µm spherical aberration

Complete wavefront

Total RMS error 0.46 µm

Fig. 5: Wavefront total results

Table 1: Zernike polynomials up to the forth order

Term	Polar representation	Monomial representation	Meaning
$Z_0(x,y)$	1	1	Constant term
$Z_1(x,y)$	rsenq	x	Tilt on x direction
$Z_2(x,y)$	rconsq	y	Tilt on y direction
$Z_3(x,y)$	r^2sen(2q)	2xy	Astigmatism with axis at $\pm45°$
$Z_4(x,y)$	$2r^2 - 1$	$-1 + 2y^2 + 2x^2$	Focal aberration (myopia or hyperopia)
$Z_5(x,y)$	r^2cos(2q)	$y^2 - x^2$	Astigmatism with axis at $\pm90°$
$Z_6(x,y)$	r^3sen(3q)	$3xy^2 - x^3$	
$Z_7(x,y)$	$(3r^3 - 2p)$senq	$-2x + 3xy^2 + 3x^3$	Coma of 3rd order at x axis
$Z_8(x,y)$	$(3r^3 - 2p)$cosq	$-2y + 3y^3 + 3x^2y$	Coma of 3rd order at y axis
$Z_9(x,y)$	r^3cos(3q)	$y^3 - 3x^2y$	
$Z_{10}(x,y)$	r^4sen(4q)	$4y^3x - 4x^3y$	
$Z_{11}(x,y)$	$(4r^4 - 3r^2)$sen(2q)	$-6xy + 8y^3x + 8x^3y$	
$Z_{12}(x,y)$	$6r^4 - 6r^2 + 1$	$1 - 6y^2 - 6x^2 + 6y^4 + 12x^2y^2 - 6x^4$	Spherical aberration of 3rd order
$Z_{13}(x,y)$	$(4r^4 - 3r^2) + cos(2q)$	$-3y^2 + 3x^2 + 4y^4 - 4x^2y^2 - 4x^4$	
$Z_{14}(x,y)$	r^4cos(4q)	$y^4 - 6x^2y^2 + x^4$	

We will discuss the Hartman-Shack aberrometer because it is the most popular instrument used in the clinical practice. The concept of H-S that a narrow beam from monochromatic light source (the laser diode) was collimated and delivered to the eye which projects a light spot on the retina, part of the light is reflected back from the point source. Because the shape of an aberrated wavefront surface changes as it propagates, the exit pupil of the eye is imaged to the lenslet array of the CCD camera by a set of relay lenses. The wavefront aberrations at the exit pupil of the eye are then measured as shown in the following image.

In perfect eye, the reflected plane wave will be focused into images with each point locating on the optical axis of the corresponding lenslet, otherwise the aberrated wavefront shows a distorted grid pattern. By measuring the displacement of each point from its corresponding lenslet axis, the slope of aberrated wavefront when it entered the lenslet can be calculated. After mathematical integration of the slope, the final aberration map will be obtained then the measured wavefront aberrations can be described and analyzed with the earlier introduced Zernike polynomials **(Figs 6 to 8)**.

Metrics to Define Image Quality

Root Mean Square Aberration

It is a measure of the magnitude of the wave aberrations. In another words, the root mean square aberration (RMS) is the standard deviation of total wavefront with respect to ideal. The RMS calculated as the square root of the sum of the square of the Zernike coefficients. The following equation shows such a calculation:

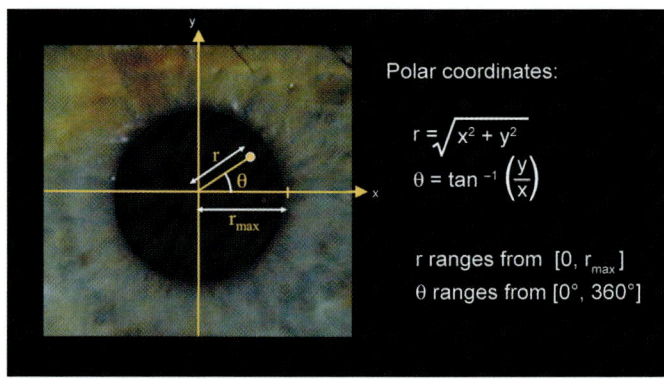

Fig. 6: Zernike pupil related

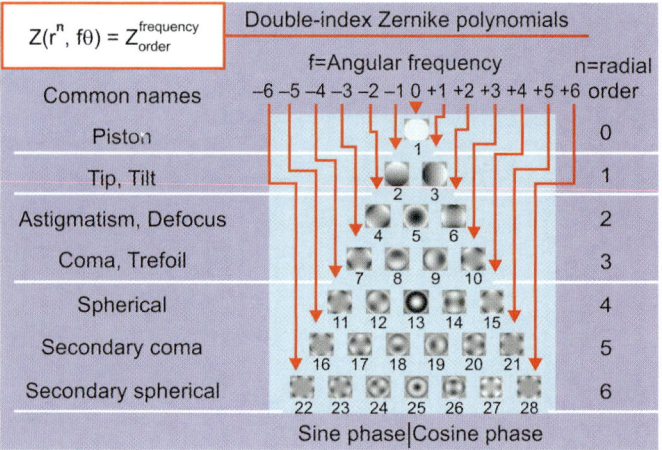

Fig. 7: Zernike index

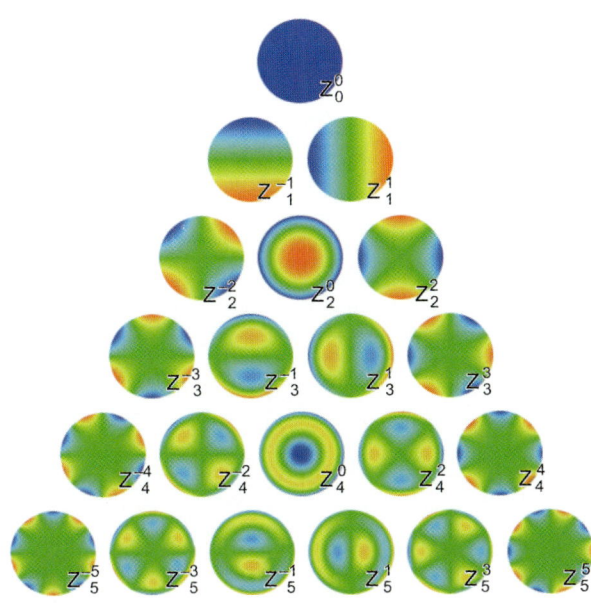

Fig. 8: Zernike images

$$RMS = \sqrt{Z^{-2}_2 + Z^0_2 + Z^2_2 + Z^{-3}_3} + \dots$$

RMS error has limited utility as an ideal single metric for visual performance because it does not show how a given aberration affects visual performance.

Point Spread Function

Objects are made up of an infinite number of points. The point spread function (PSF) of the eye describes how each object point is imaged on the retina. Consequently the PSF is one of the fundamental methods for describing the optical quality of an imaging system such as the eye. So in a perfect optical system, the PSF should look like a point or a distant star **(Figs 9 to 12)**.

Strehl Ratio

Before we talk about this ratio, we must clarify what do we mean by DIFFRACTION. Diffraction is defined as deviation of the light rays from rectilinear path that cannot be interpreted as reflection or refraction. Diffraction effects are pupil size dependent. The diffraction effects induced by the pupil diameter are easily viewed by observing how increasing pupil diameter decrease diameter of the PSF in a perfect eye (no wavefront aberrations—such an optical system is often referred to as diffraction limited).

The Strehl ratio is measurement correlated for PSF. It expresses the relationship between the real luminous intensity of the object-image and the maximum intensity of a focal point limited by diffraction alone.

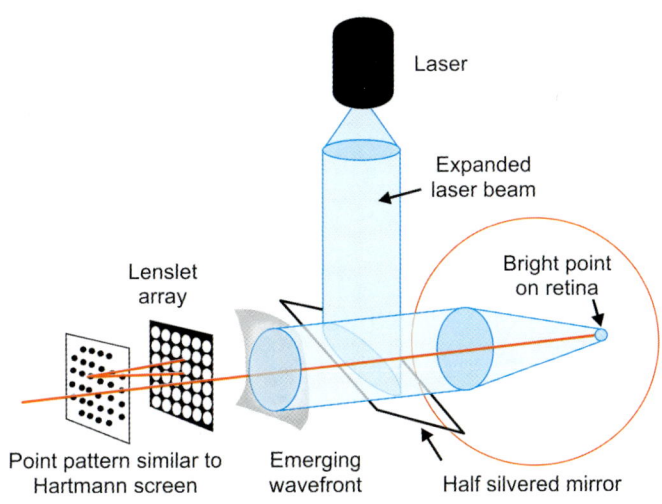

Fig. 9: Point patterns

In another words, the Strehl ratio is the ratio between the peak heights of the PSF over the peak height for the same optical system if it were diffraction limited (dl) **(Fig. 13)**.

Modulation Transfer Function

The modulation transfer function (MTF) indicates the ability of an optical system to reproduce (transfer) various levels of detail (spatial frequencies) from the object to the image. Its units are the ratio of image contrast over the object contrast as a function of spatial frequency.

A person, for example is composed of many spatial frequencies from low (torso, arms, legs) to high (facial features, hair, etc.). We all know that fine detail or high spatial frequencies are the first to be get lost when you degrade an image. When you are out of focus, you can still make out a person (low spatial frequencies), but you may not identify his or her fine facial features (high spatial frequencies).

Phase Transfer Function

When spatial frequencies get transferred to the image plane, the location of the bright and dark bars, called the PHASE of the reduced–contrast grating may also be shifted. In another words, it is the phase difference between the object image and retinal image.

Optical Transfer Function

The MTF and the phase transfer function (PTF) combine to form the optical transfer function (OTF). Like the PSF, the OTF is an entirely adequate and complete way to present how an image is formed by the optical system. In the simple words, in a healthy visual system, the improvement in the quality of

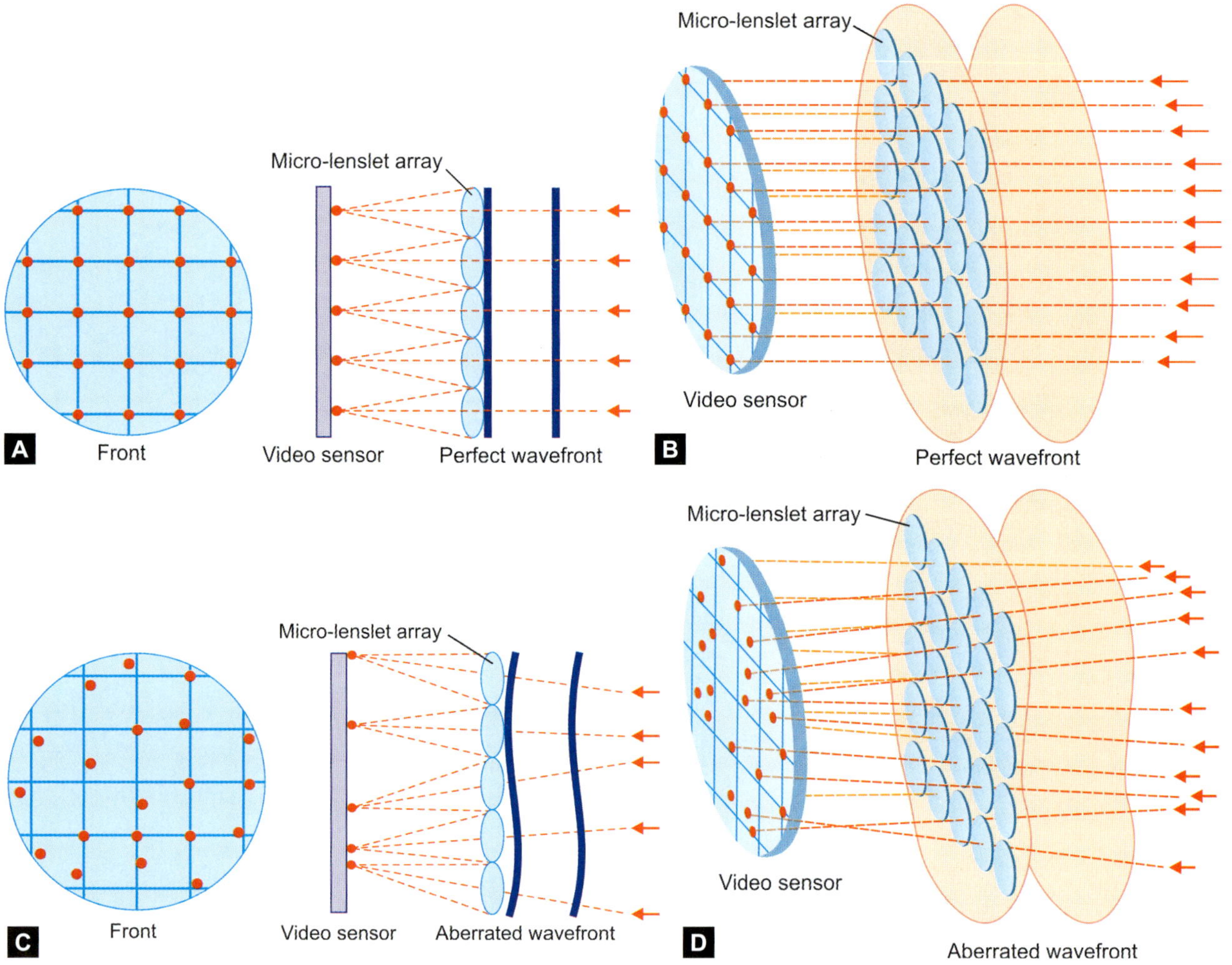

Micro-lenslet array
A
Front
Video sensor
Perfect wavefront
Micro-lenslet array
B
Video sensor
Perfect wavefront
Micro-lenslet array
C
Front
Video sensor
Aberrated wavefront
Micro-lenslet array
D
Video sensor
Aberrated wavefront

Figs 10A to D: Process from perfect to aberrated wavefront

1 mm
2 mm
3 mm
4 mm
5 mm
6 mm
7 mm

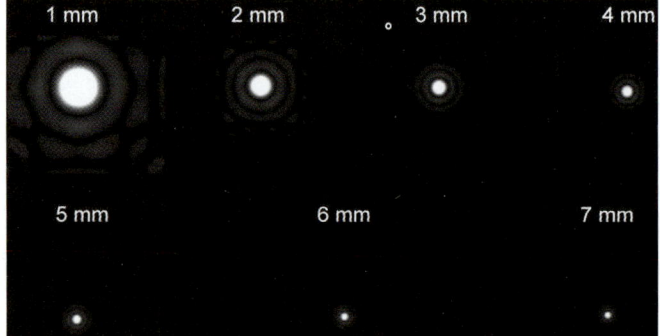

Fig. 11: PSF for increasing pupil sizes in perfect eye, the small pupil size as 1 mm. The image-point is large due to diffraction not aberrations

1 mm
2 mm
3 mm
4 mm
5 mm
6 mm
7 mm

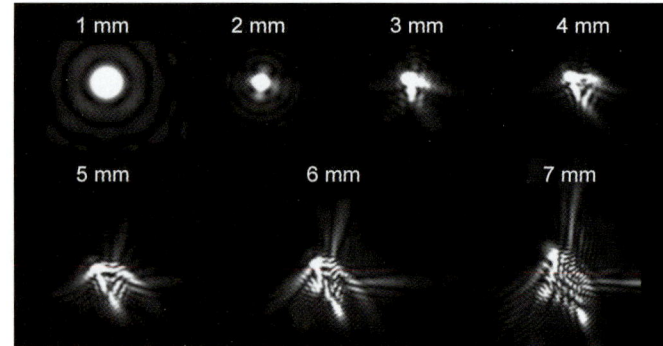

Fig. 12: PSF of increasing pupil sizes in a typical human eye, the effect of aberrations as the pupil size increase is very obvious

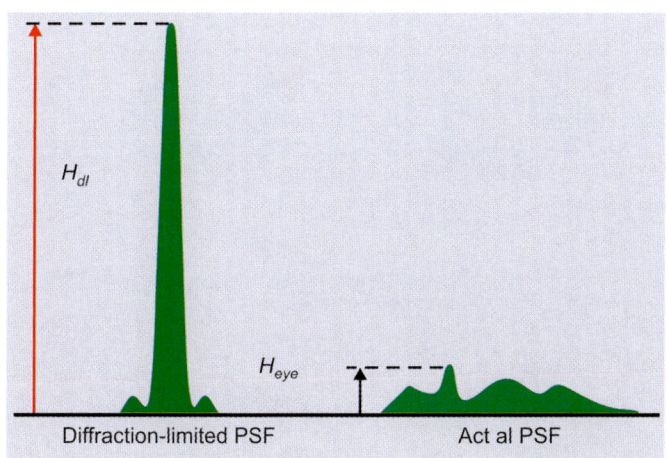

Fig. 13: Pictorial definition of Strehl ratio. The maximum value of Strehl ratio is 1, which occurs when the optical system is diffraction limited

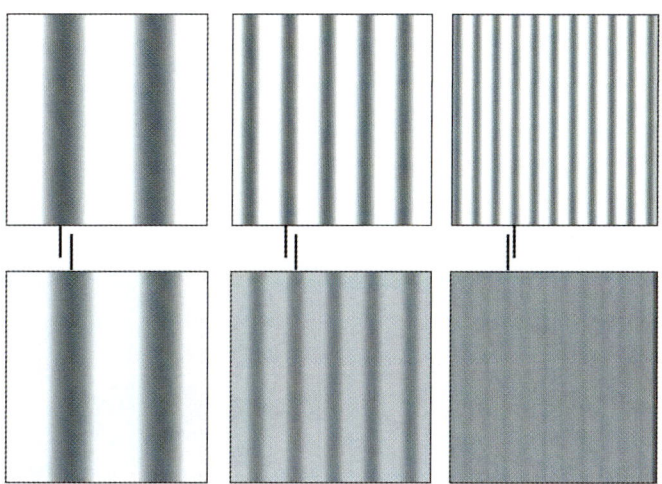

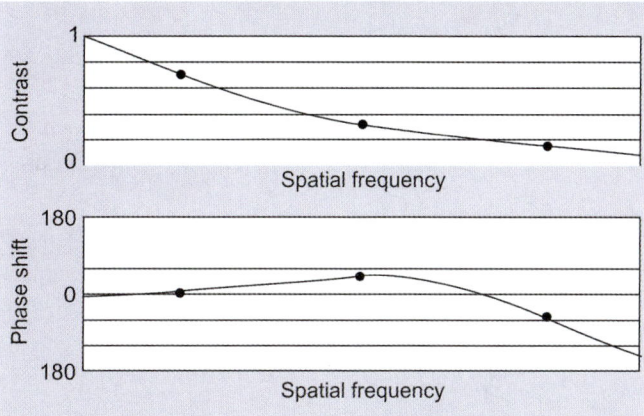

Fig. 14: Pictorial demonstration of the calculation of the MTF and the PTF. The first row shows the object, which are 100% contrast vertical sinusoidal gratings with low, medium, and high spatial frequencies. After passing through the imaging system, the gratings have less contrast and the peak locations (phase) are shifted. The MTF plots the change in contrast relative to the original object. The PTF plots the change in phase of the same grating. This procedure may be different for each orientation of the gratings. The OTF is the combination of the MTF and the PTF for all grating orientations

the retinal image is translated into greater contrast (with an increase in the MTF) and sharper definition (with reduction in PTF) **(Fig. 14)**.

Relationships Between Wavefront Aberrations, Point Spread Function and Optical Transfer Function

The wavefront aberration, the PSF, and the OTF are all intimately related. Once the wave aberration is known the PSF and OTF can be calculated. The relationships between the three are typically through the Fourier transform (Fourier transform is mathematical operation has allowed various measures of optical quality to be linked and allows the computation of the expected retinal image for any visual object). From wave aberration to PSF, one takes the Fourier transform of the complex pupil function. The OTF is the Fourier transform of the PSF.

Factors Affecting Wavefront Aberrations in the Human Eye

1. **Pupil size:** In smaller pupil size (less than 2.0 mm), diffraction affects the image quality more than aberrations. A larger pupil will allow the light rays to enter the eye through the periphery which may cause an increase of wavefront aberrations. As the pupil size increases, the effect of aberrations on image quality increases and become more dominant in the larger pupil.
2. **Accommodation:** Accommodation-induced changes of aberrations including changes of defocus, astigmatism, and high order aberrations especially the spherical aberrations which change in direction to negative with increase accommodation.
3. **Age:** The normal aging process affects all ocular tissues and causes changes to both neural and optical parameters of the human eye. Increase in the wavefront aberrations have been found in aged eyes and these changes in the ocular aberrations may be contributed by the age-related changes of two major optical components, the cornea and the crystalline lens.
4. **Refractive error:** There is conflicting results of the impact of refractive errors on the optical structure and the higher order aberrations of the eye.
5. **Ocular disease especially keratoconus:** Significant amount of corneal and ocular HOAs are induced by the

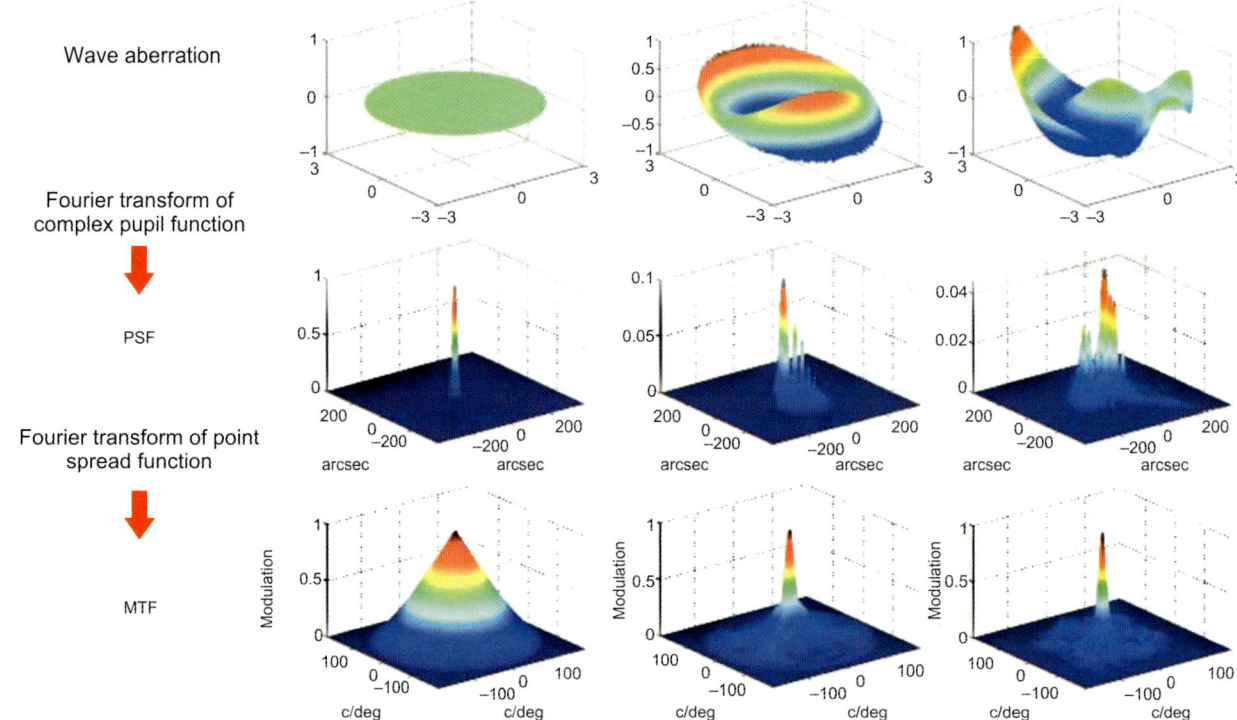

Fig. 15: Wavefront aberration, PSF and MTF for three different wave aberrations. The relation between them: when aberrations are present, the PSF broadens and becomes more irregular. The MTF shows that with aberrations, contrast drops quickly and in nonuniform manner for all high spatial frequencies

distortion of cornea in keratoconus compared to normal eyes. Coma, trefoil and spherical aberration were found to be the most dominant HOAs in both corneal and ocular aberrations in keratoconus eyes.

6. **Corneal refractive procedures:** There is induction of HOAs in many refractive procedures like PRK and LASIK.

Application of Wavefront Technology

1. **Wavefront-guided ablation:** The use of wavefront aberrometry to guide an excimer laser ablation is based on the notable theoretical advantage of correcting not only spherocylindrical errors but also the HOAs while minimizing the induction of aberrations by the laser ablation.

2. **Diagnostic and intraocular lens design applications:** The applications of wavefront sensing go far beyond wavefront-guided ablations.
   - *Diagnostic:* Wavefront technology as a diagnostic tool has been important in understanding the relationship between anatomical structures, optics, and subjective visual quality. It is necessary to diagnose visual symptoms related to aberrations such as diplopia, halos, glare as this can help determine the best treatment.
   - *Intraocular lens design:* The use of aspheric IOLs to reduce preoperative normal corneal positive spherical aberration has been shown to increase the contrast sensitivity in mesopic conditions. Customization of the selection of an IOL is a new concept that goes further than achieving emmetropia after cataract surgery. The objective is to estimate the optimum amount of spherical aberration within the eye and the IOL to optimize optical quality. The corneal HOAs are measured and help determine the best IOL according to the expected induction in spherical aberration. Appropriate IOL selection is becoming more important as more patients with prior refractive surgery are now in need of cataract extraction.

3. **Expanding the depth of focus by modifying higher-order aberrations:** Although HOAs degrade the quality of vision in most circumstances, in some instances they

may have a beneficial effect. In the case of presbyopia, the induction of specific HOAs may expand the depth of focus without significantly compromising the quality of vision and this will improve the near vision with compromising the distant vision **(Fig. 15)**.

CONCLUSION

Wavefront technology is a new tool that will have a widespread application in the field of ophthalmology so every ophthalmologist must have a good insight about this subject.

BIBLIOGRAPHY

1. Borish's clinical refraction, 2nd edn. Chapter 19 (wavefront refraction).
2. Mello GR, Rocha KM, Santhiago MR, et al. Applications of wavefront technology. J Cataract Refract Surg. 2012;38:1671-83.
3. Wavefront customized visual correction. The Quest for Supervision 2 Slack Incorporated. 2004.

CHAPTER **6**

Vance Thompson

Basic Wavefront Optics and Ocular Aberrations

INTRODUCTION

The surgical treatment of refractive error involves precision preoperative measurements. For decades, the phoropter has been a critical tool for measuring refractive error. A traditional phoropter or loose lens refraction will measure spherical and regular astigmatism refractive error only. For many patients, this is enough for quality vision but for some it may not be. For any doctor that has diligently performed a manifest refraction for an otherwise healthy patient with a seemingly healthy ocular system, it can be frustrating when the patient feels that even though they can read the 20/20 line the letters look 'fuzzy' or have a 'ghost image'. Prior to this century, even though we knew that internal high order aberrations were often the culprit blurring retinal image quality, we had no technology to document this. We called refractive error that we could not correct with a refraction, for lack of a better term, irregular astigmatism.

Wavefront technology allowed us, for the first time in history, to diagnostically measure beyond regular sphere and cylinder, which allowed us to clinically understand the low and high order aberration state of an eye and thus start to define much more specifically these high order terms, we had been calling irregular astigmatism.[1-3] In a short period of time, wavefront testing of eyes has revolutionized the definition of refractive error.[4] Wavefront measuring devices, also known as aberrometers, have allowed us the ability to measure and subsequently both quantify and mathematically describe these aberrations so that these more accurate measurements could be used to develop treatment plans that would drive the excimer laser for ablation patterns that addressed low order aberrations in smaller increments that was ever before possible plus describe and treat for the first time ever, the patients high order aberrations.[5]

WAVEFRONT TECHNOLOGY IN CLINICAL PRACTICE

In wavefront terminology low order aberrations (LOAs) refer to myopia, hyperopia, and astigmatism. In an otherwise healthy eye, LOAs make the vast majority of refractive error and high order aberrations (HOAs) make up a much smaller portion or the total error. Wavefront technology allows the examiner to learn much more about the optical state of a patient's eye **(Fig. 1)**. If there is pathology such as corneal trauma, previous corneal surgery (refractive or therapeutic), significant dry eye, corneal edema, or anything else besides a normal cornea the amount of HOAs can become large enough to be a significant cause of visual blur or frustration[6-9] **(Figs 2 and 3)**. Reduced image quality, glare, and halos from elevated HOAs can be measured, quantified, and potentially treated. It is also important to realize that HOAs can be very normal and be present in eyes with very good vision **(Figs 4A and B)**. HOA patterns can also share certain characteristics in certain disease states like keratoconus.[10] Wavefront analysis can tell us vital information in laser vision correction patients

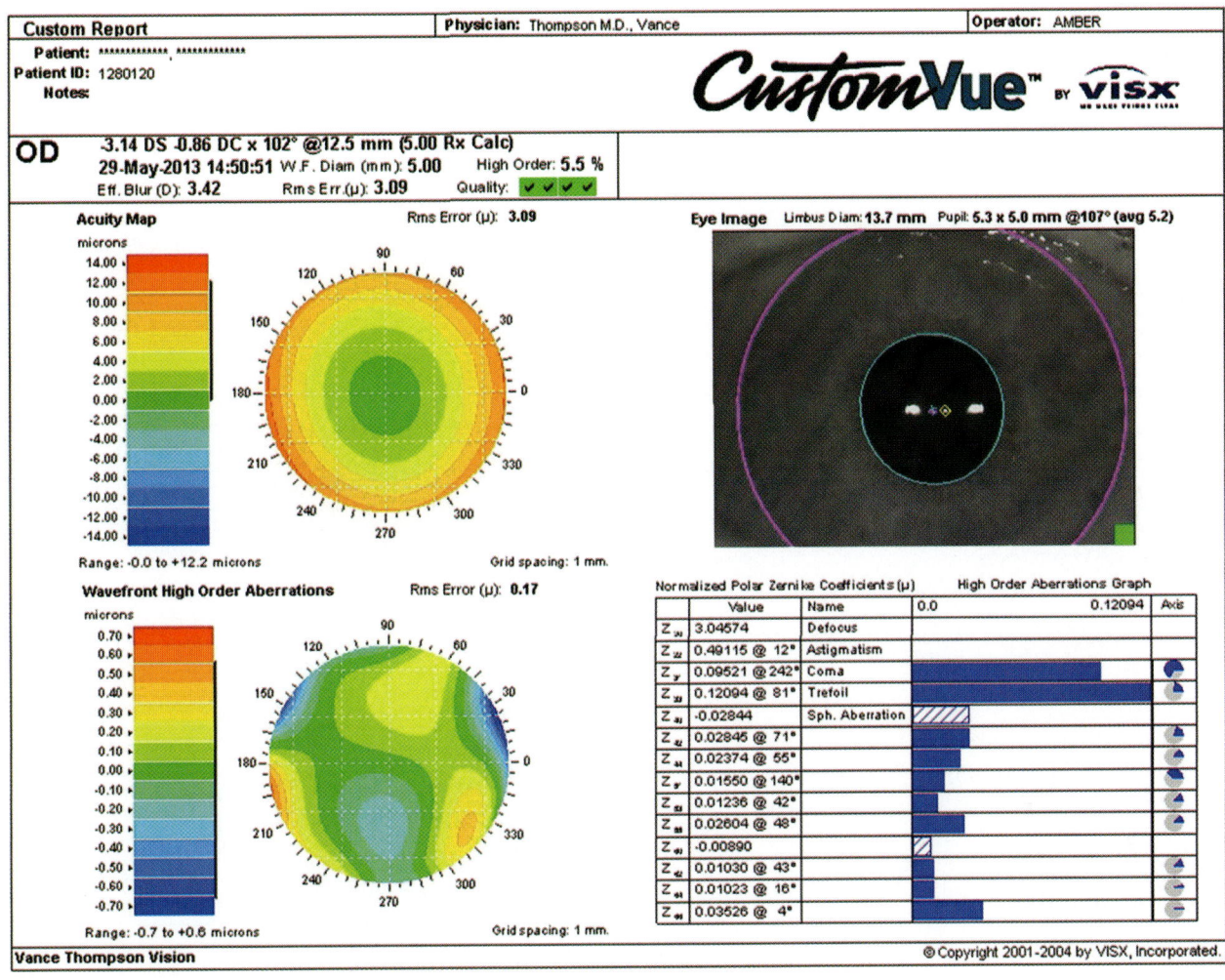

Fig. 1: Wavefront analysis provides much more data than manifest refraction. This 55-year-old preoperative wavefront shows HOAs of 5.4% and a detailed analysis of both a wavefront derived LOA refraction and breakdown and magnitude of HOAs

with a near plano result but still not satisfied with their image quality **(Figs 5A and B)**. This data can then be used to develop vision changing treatment plans that can help these frustrated patients achieve a quality visual result. Finally, wavefront changes occur naturally with aging, such as an increase in spherical aberration due to lenticular changes with time, and it is important to take these changes into consideration when analyzing aberration maps[11,12] **(Figs 6 and 7)**. That is why, it is important to learn wavefront technology and apply it to the overall clinical situation when trying to decide whether HOAs need to be addressed surgically, optically, or not.

In the world of wavefront terminology, myopia and hyperopia are referred to as defocus. Defocus and astigmatism are called 2nd order aberrations **(Fig. 8)**. Measuring defocus and astigmatism is most commonly done with a phoropter or autorefractor. High order aberrations (HOAs) comprise a variety of aberrations with names such as coma, trefoil, and spherical aberration.

WAVEFRONT MEASURING DEVICES: ABERROMETERS

There are many more HOAs and the measurement of them with what is called an aberrometer requires more sophisticated techniques such as Shack-Hartmann sensing can provide data from which the wave aberrations of the human eye can be accurately and reliably quantified **(Fig. 9)**. Clinical aberrometers provide very detailed measurements of the eye's wavefront aberration state and have become very important in modern day eyecare both diagnostically and for optical and surgical treatment planning. The total

2 SECTION

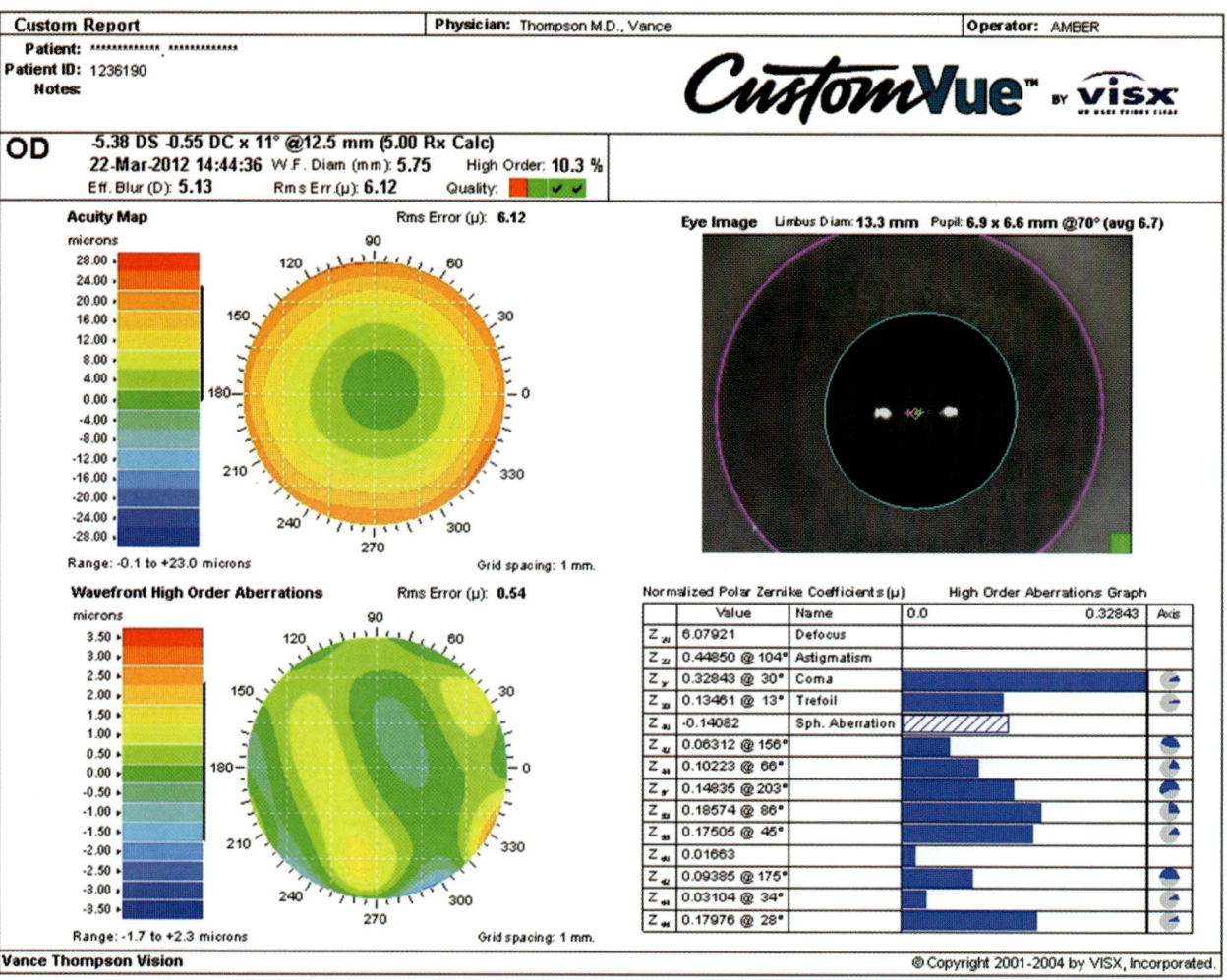

Fig. 2A: Dry eye can significantly impact a wavefront due to tear film irregularities inducting high order aberrations as shown in on the left in this 32-year-old preoperative LASIK with newly diagnosed dry eye

wavefront error and the individual contribution of each higher-order aberration in the individual eye can now be accurately determined and quantified by these aberrometers. An aberrometer is basically a wavefront sensing device which measures the wavefront as it exits the eye. They can only analyze data that comes through the pupil so typically having a dilated pupil for the examination is helpful, but not always necessary, to assess pupillary areas used in low light situations. Accommodation should be controlled for, ideally with cylcoplegia. Any dry eye should be treated also since an irregular tear film can cause unpredictable changes in the wavefront and make the measurement less accurate.[6-8]

As stated previously a common aberrometer used in clinical practice is the Hartmann-Shack aberrometer. This technology works by projected a highly collimated light source onto the retina which then reflects off the retina, comes back through the lens, through the pupil, and exits the eye through the cornea. This wavefront is then focused by individual lenses called lenslets. This array of lenslets in the aberrometer each have the same focal length. Each is focused onto a photosensor (typically CCD). In this way, a very detailed analysis across the entire wavefront occurs with the final result being a quite accurate (but not perfect) reconstruction of the patient's total (LOAs and HOAs) optical data. There are other wavefront

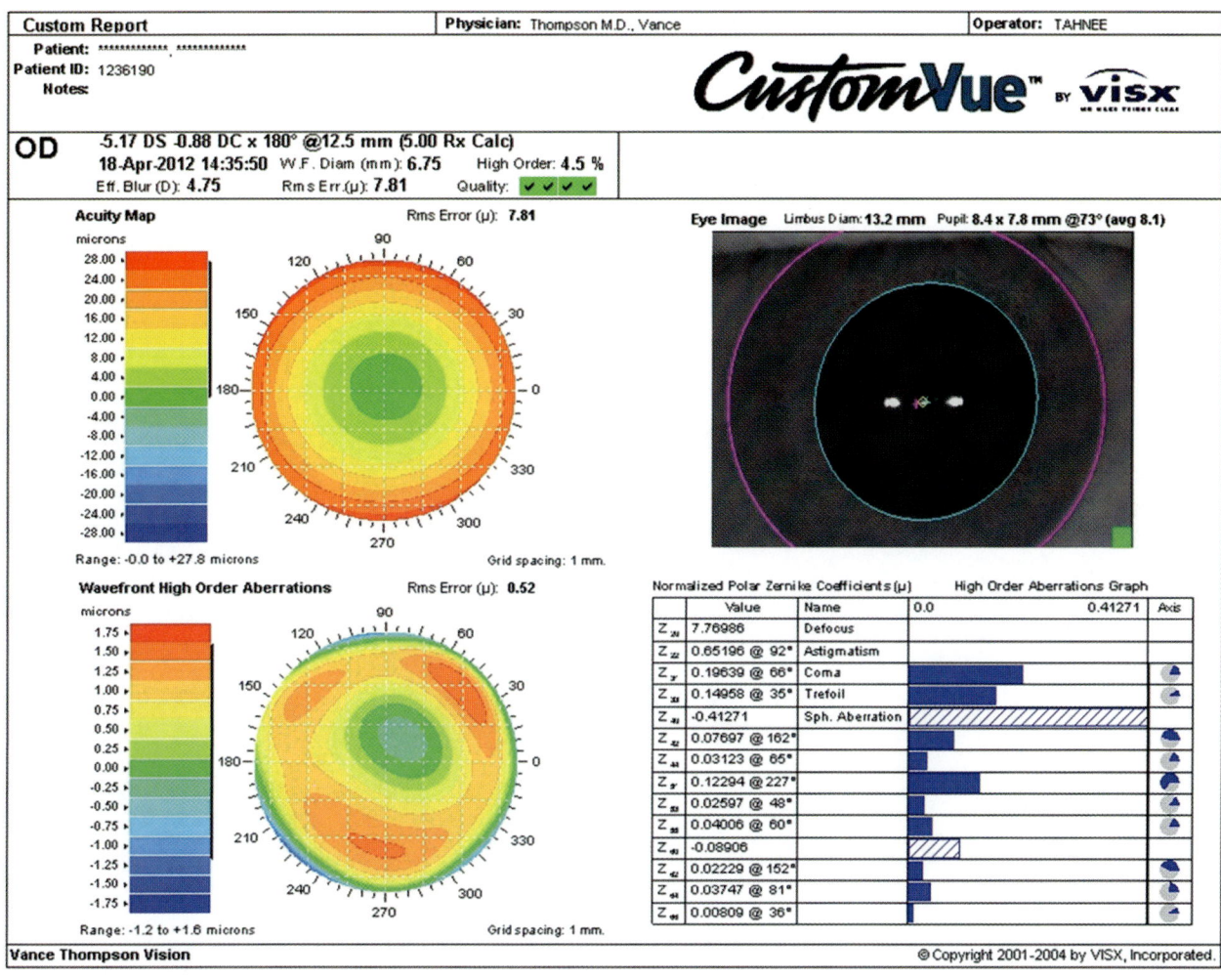

Fig. 2B: With 4 weeks of dry eye therapy, this same dry eye patient the wavefront is much improved with lower HOAs and a better quality wavefront

analyzers used clinically also. The construction of a wavefront map utilizes sophisticated mathematics called polynomials to describe it in details that allow it to be clinically useful and put into color maps that share similarities with corneal topography for helpful viewing.[3,13]

ANALYSIS OF THE WAVEFRONT DATA

As mentioned above, the shape of a wavefront is mathematically described complex equations called polynomials.[13-16] A common mathematical method used to describe these measured LOAs and HOAs is Zernike or Fourier polynomials.[3,17,18] They share many similarities but also differences that are beyond the goals of this chapter. The main purpose in this discussion is to understand that after a clinical wavefront sensing device captures wavefront data exiting an eye these mathematical polynomial equations are used to describe the wavefront numerically or graphically. This data is able to describe both wavefront aberrations and corneal surfaces and thus be used diagnostically to assess the overall optical quality of an eye plus design customized corneal ablations for PRK or LASIK.[19,20]

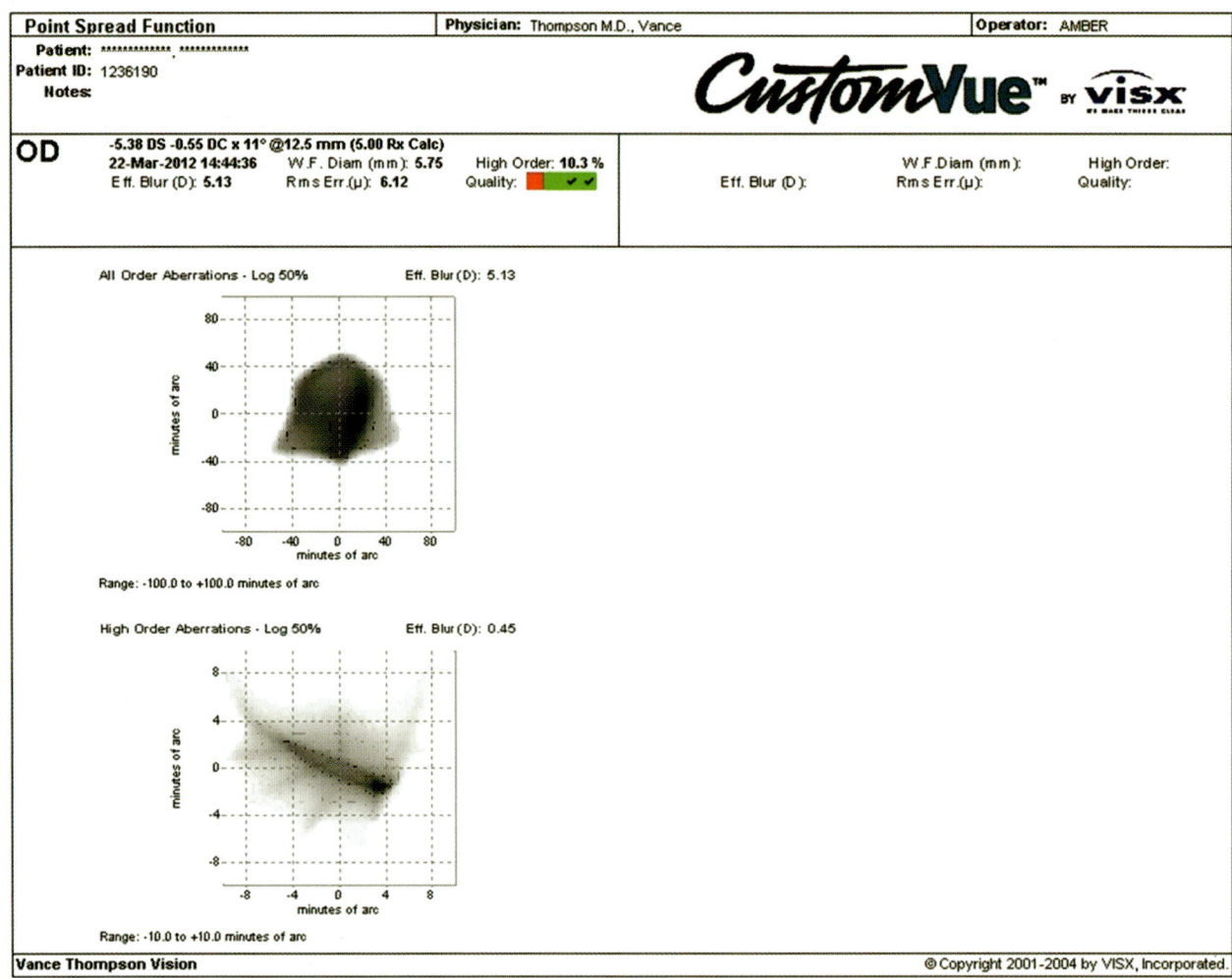

| Point Spread Function | Physician: Thompson M.D., Vance | | Operator: AMBER |

Patient: ＊＊＊＊＊＊＊＊＊＊＊＊ ＊＊＊＊＊＊＊＊＊＊＊＊
Patient ID: 1236190
Notes:

CustomVue™ by **visx**

OD
-5.38 DS -0.55 DC x 11° @12.5 mm (5.00 Rx Calc)
22-Mar-2012 14:44:36   W.F. Diam (mm): 5.75   High Order: 10.3 %
E ff. Blur (D): 5.13   Rms Err.(μ): 6.12   Quality: ✔ ✔

Eff. Blur (D):   W.F.Diam (mm):   High Order:
Rms Err.(μ):   Quality:

All Order Aberrations - Log 50%   Eff. Blur (D): 5.13

Range: -100.0 to +100.0 minutes of arc

High Order Aberrations - Log 50%   Eff. Blur (D): 0.45

Range: -10.0 to +10.0 minutes of arc

Vance Thompson Vision   © Copyright 2001-2004 by VISX, Incorporated.

Fig. 3A: Point spread function (PSF) of the same 32-year-old preoperative LASIK patient in
Figure 2 on the left in this with newly diagnosed dry eye

A common clinically useful way to describe the wavefront shape uses a single number to describe the amount the wavefront deviates from a plane wave called the root mean square (RMS) error.[3,21] Mathematically, it represents the standard deviation of the wavefront from a plane wave and is often used to describe the overall optical quality of the eye. The RMS can be calculated for the total aberration or for the individual higher-order aberrations (HOAs). It is important to remember that the RMS value is a number that indicates the magnitude of the aberration but not its unique shape. A perfect optical system would have a flat wavefront and an RMS of zero. Evaluating root mean square (RMS) values helps us understand the optical quality of an eye. The higher the RMS value the greater the number of aberrations. Typically, patients who have fewer total aberrations (lower RMS value) tend to have better contrast sensitivity and low light image quality. A perfect example of this is comparing **Figure 4** where the 22-year-old patient has quality vision and an HOA-RMS value of 0.18 while the 27-year-old with glare and halos in **Figure 5** has an RMS value of 0.94.

Wavefront analysis gives other important parameters helpful in analyzing a patient's image quality, namely, point spread function (PSF) and modulation transfer function (MTF).[19] The PSF image is formed by light from a point source

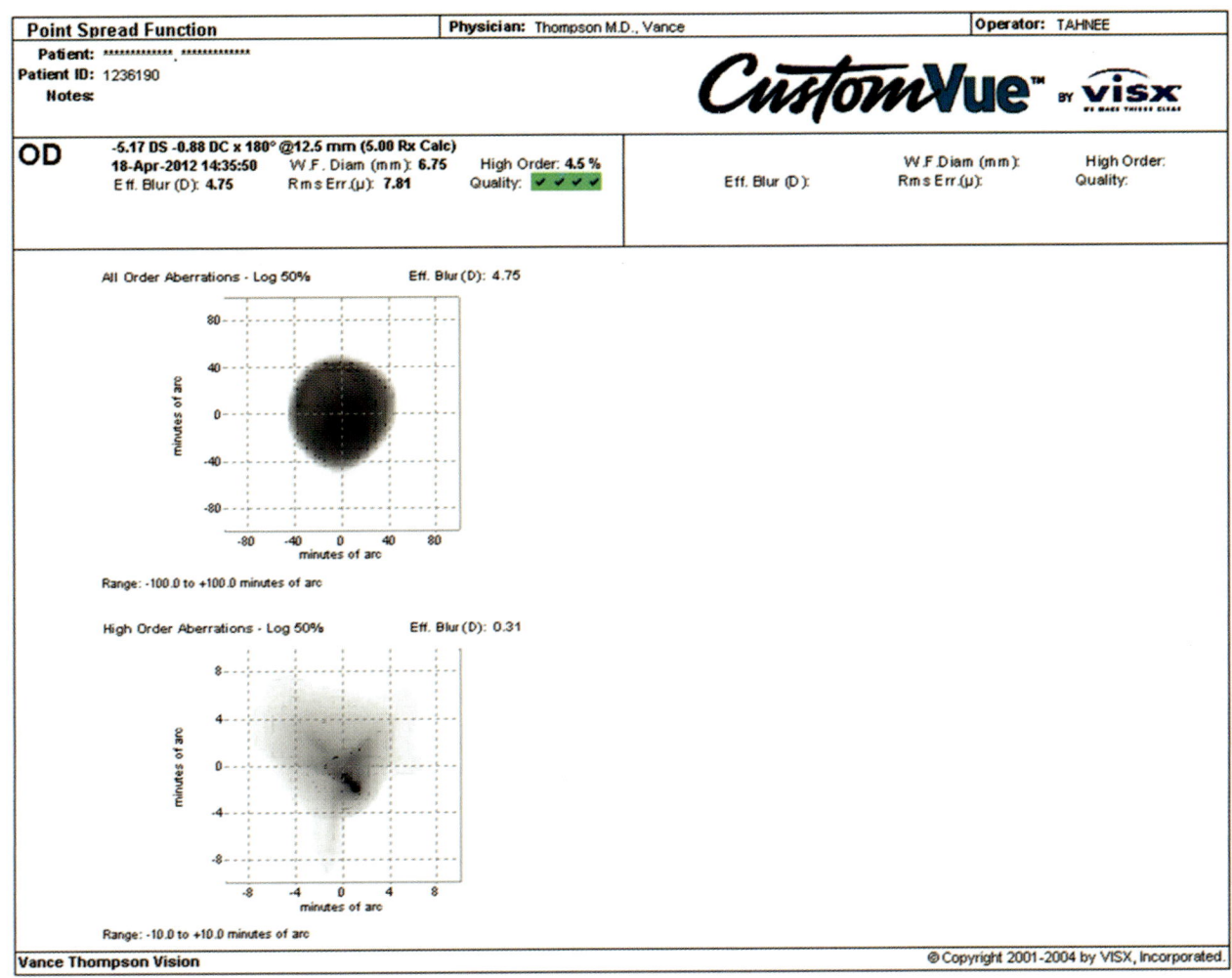

Fig. 3B: With 4 weeks of dry eye therapy, this same dry eye patient the point spread function is much improved with lower HOAs and a better quality wavefront

traveling through an optical system. The PSF is small and highly focused in an eye with minimal aberrations **(Fig. 4)**. The PSF is large, irregular, and highly defocused in an eye with a lot of aberrations and poor image quality **(Fig. 5)**. The MTF measures the loss of contrast with increasing spatial frequency when an image travels through an aberrated optical system. Spatial frequency refers to the number of pairs of bars imaged within a given distance on the retina and is defined by the number of cycles (line pairs) per unit distance. It is known that high spatial frequencies (fine details, closely spaced alternation black and white fine lines) are the first to be affected when the quality of an optical system is degraded. MTF quantifies this loss.

Besides looking at the low and high order aberration state of an eye, it can be very helpful clinically to routinely assess these useful parameters such as RMS, PSF, and MTF.

CONCLUSION

Understanding the total optics of the eye is critically important diagnostically and in developing surgical plans. Custom laser vision correction addressing both low and high order aberrations was made possible by wavefront technology. Wavefront technology has forever revolutionized, how we analyze the optical state of the eye.

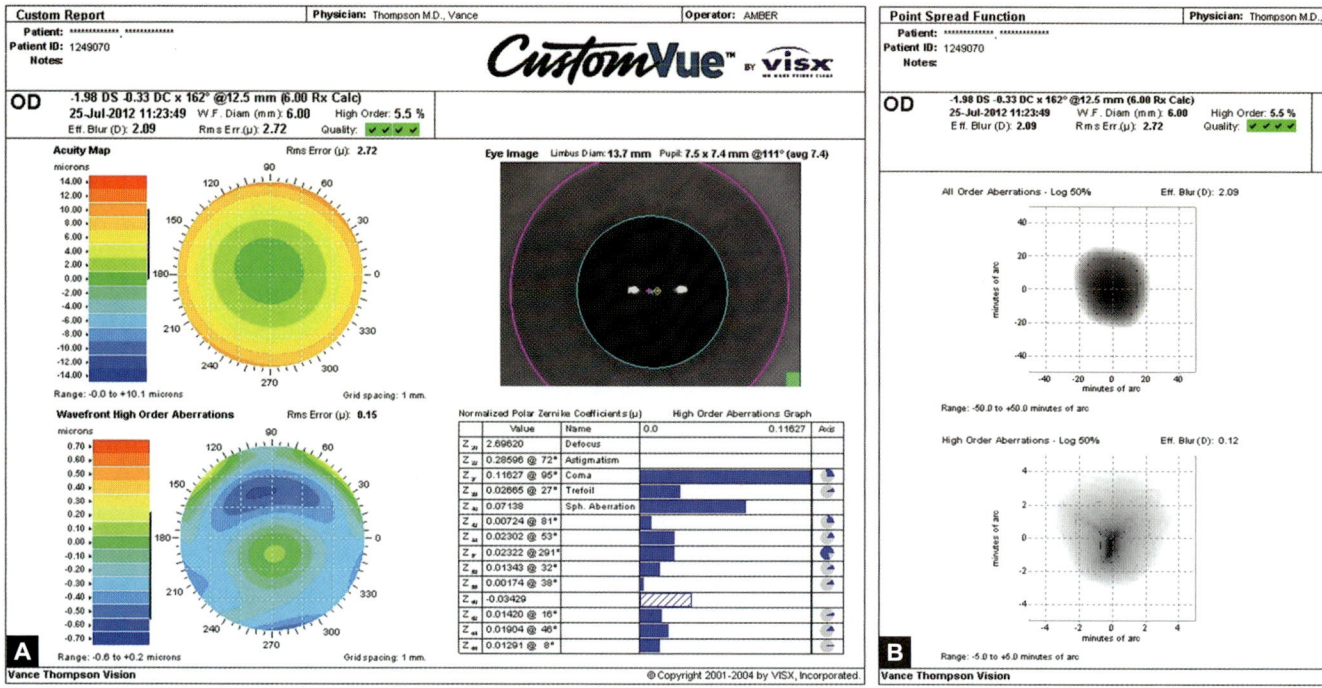

Figs 4A and B: (A) High order aberrations are present also in eyes with quality vision and no glare or halos. This is a 22-year-old patient happy with their image quality. Note HOA of 7.4%, Coma of 0.116, and spherical aberration of 0.07. (B) Point spread function of the same patient

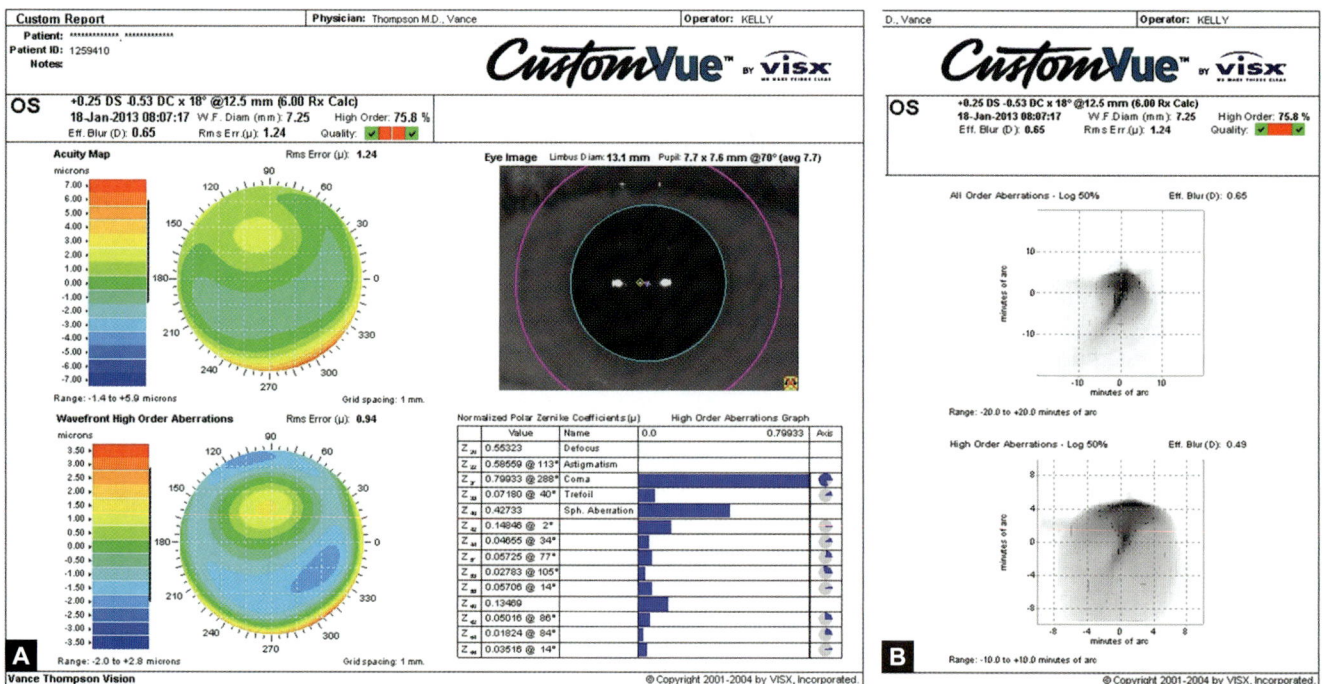

Figs 5A and B: (A) A 27-year-old post-LASIK patient who has had previous conventional treatment of myopia and sphere who suffers from glare and halos due to induced high order aberrations. Their wavefront quantifies their high and low order aberrations to aid in treatment planning. (B) Point spread function, if the same patient on the right

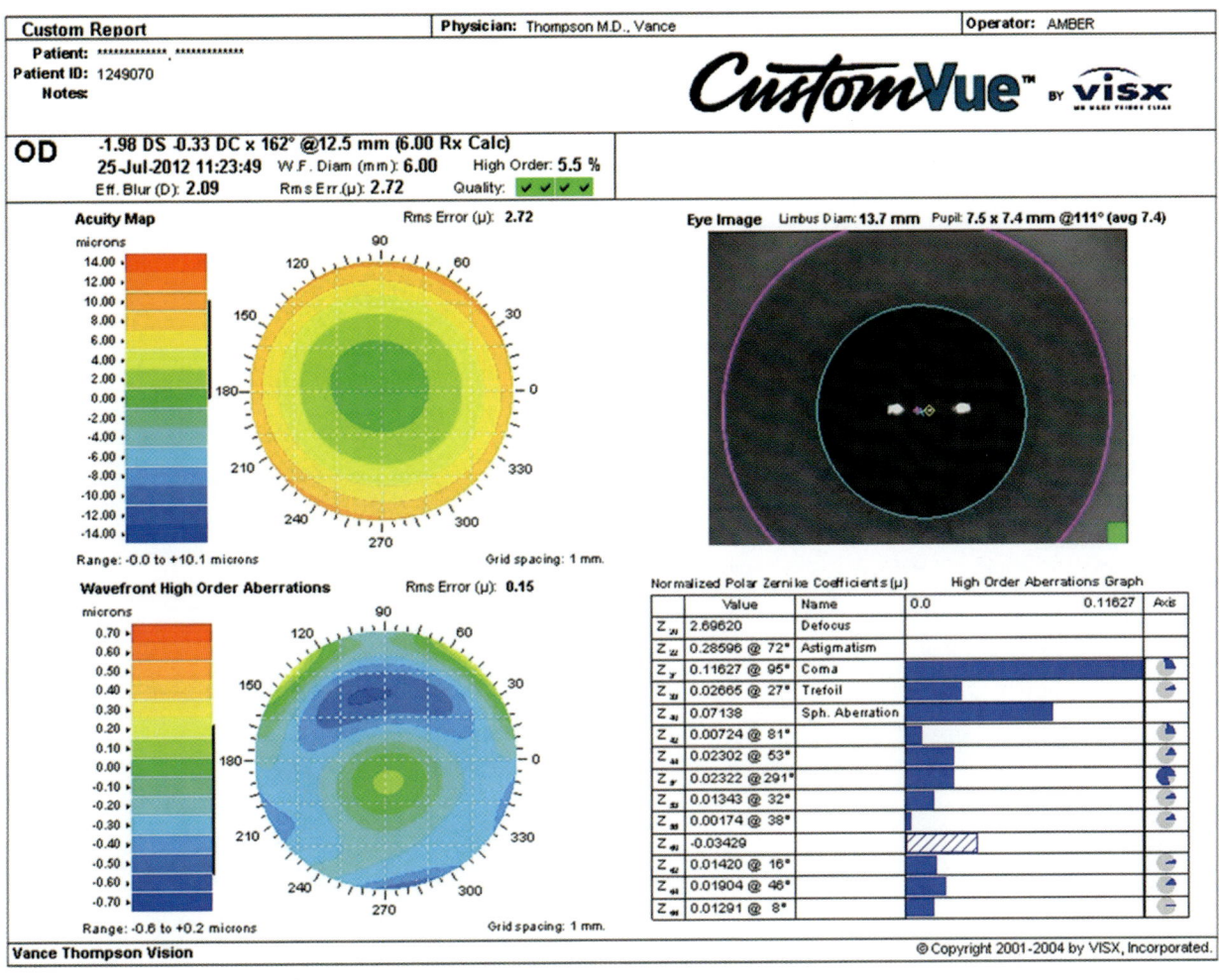

Fig. 6A: Wavefront changes normally with age. Note spherical aberration in this 22-year-old patient with 20/20 best corrected vision (BCVA) and no complaints

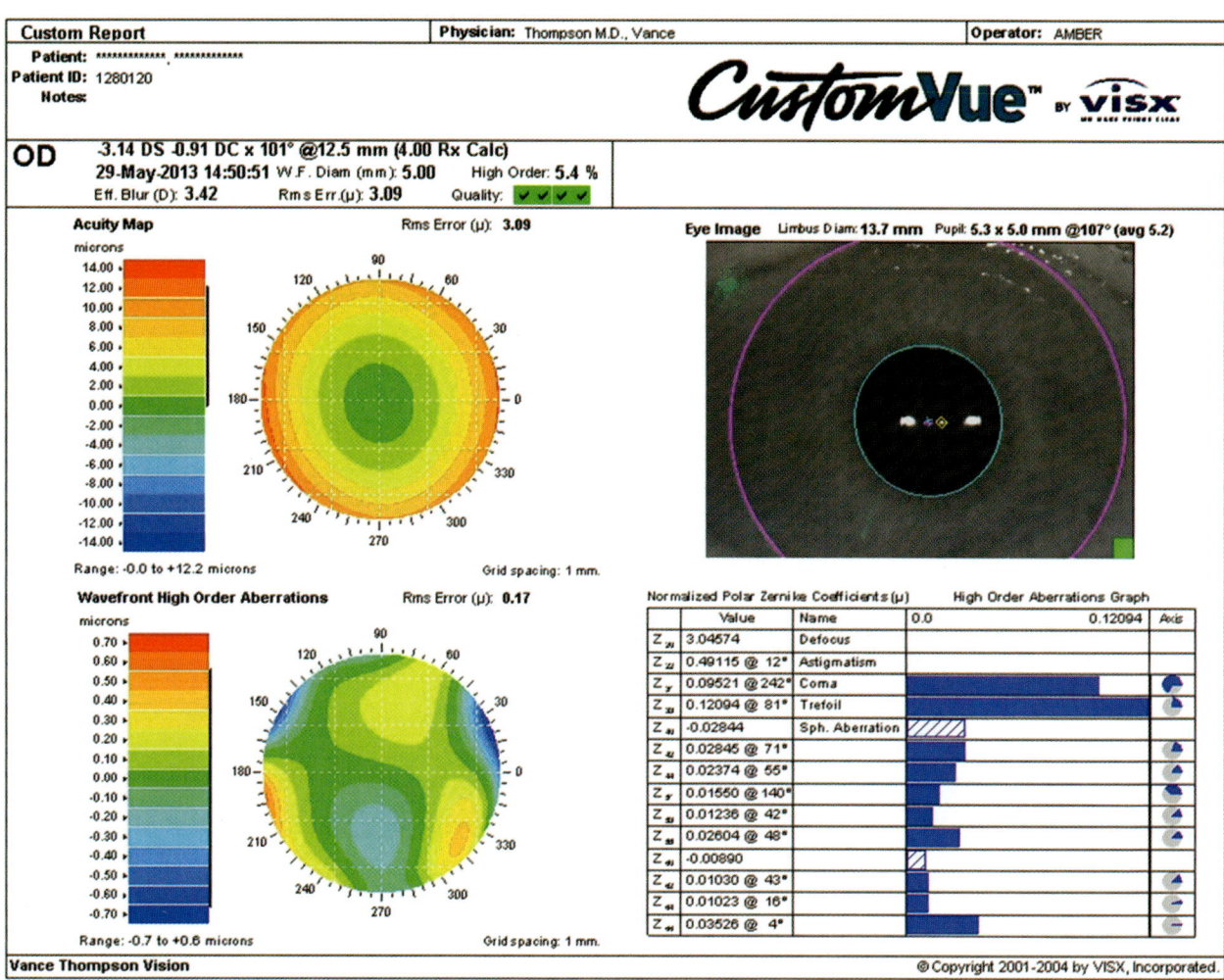

Fig. 6B: Wavefront changes normally with age. Note spherical aberration for this 53-year-old patient with 20/20 BCVA and no complaints

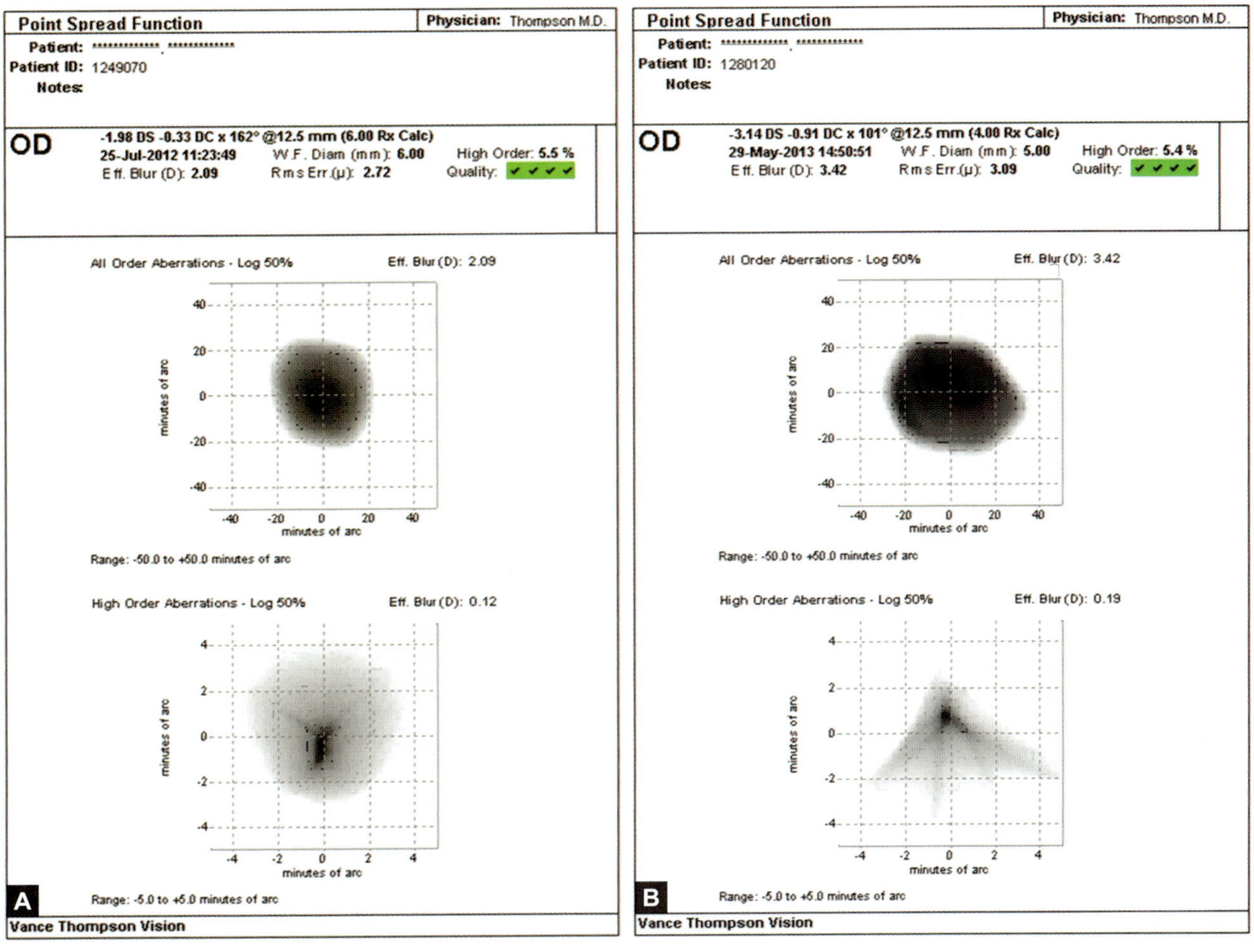

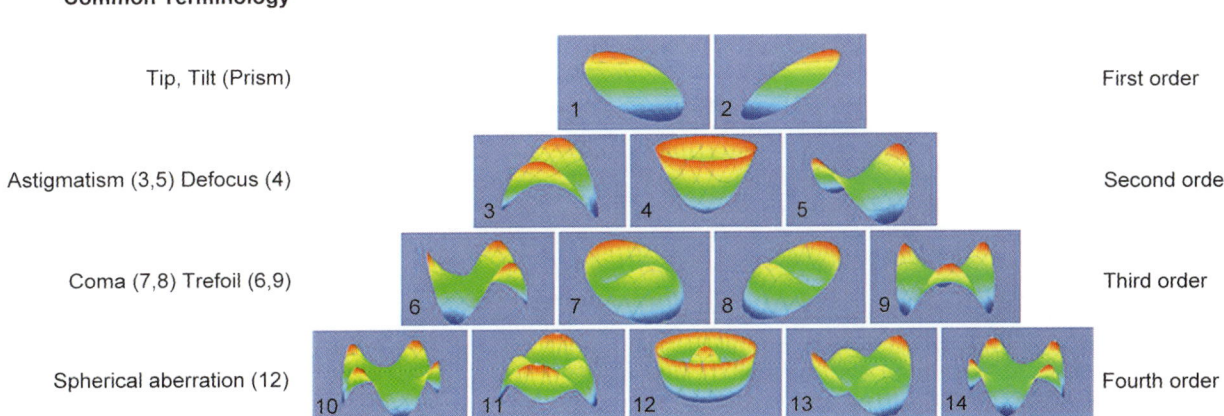

Figs 7A and B: Same patients as in Figure 6 showing how point spread function changes normally with age also. (A) Note point spread function in this 22-year-old patient with 20/20 best corrected vision (BCVA) and no complaints. (B) Note point spread function for this 53-year-old patient with 20/20 BCVA and no complaints

Common Terminology

Tip, Tilt (Prism)	First order
Astigmatism (3,5) Defocus (4)	Second order
Coma (7,8) Trefoil (6,9)	Third order
Spherical aberration (12)	Fourth order

Fig. 8: Zernike polynomials

2 SECTION

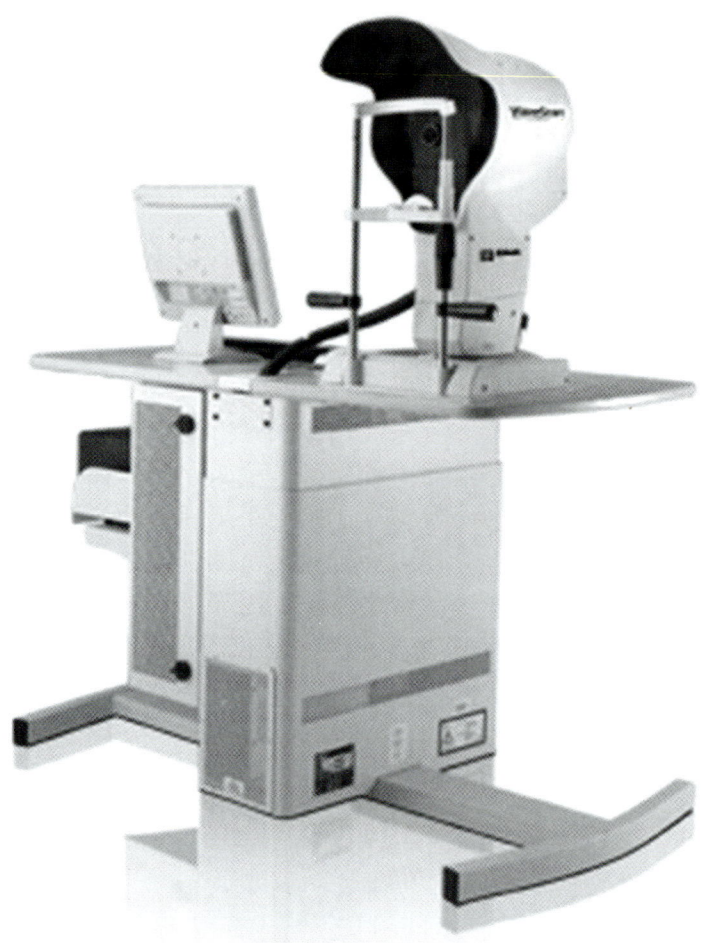

Fig. 9: The VISX WaveScan Wavefront System is an example of a common clinically used Hartmann-Shack Aberrometer. The WaveScan wavefront system uses the same Hartmann-Shack technology used in the Hubble space telescope

REFERENCES

1. Huelle JO, Katz T, Draeger J, Pahlitzsch M, Druchkiv V, Steinberg J, Richard G, Linke SJ. Accuracy of wavefront aberrometer refraction vs manifest refraction in cataract patients: impact of age, ametropia and visual function. Graefes Arch Clin Exp Ophthalmol. 2013;251(4):1163-73.
2. López-Miguel A, Martínez-Almeida L, González-García MJ, Coco-Martín MB, Sobrado-Calvo P, Maldonado MJ. Precision of higher-order aberration measurements with a new placido-disk topographer and Hartmann-Shack wavefront sensor. J Cataract Refract Surg. 2013;39(2):242-9.
3. Mello GR, Rocha KM, Santhiago MR, Smadja D, Krueger RR. Applications of wavefront technology. J Cataract Refract Surg. 2012;38(9):1671-83.
4. López-Miguel A, Maldonado MJ, Belzunce A, Barrio-Barrio J, Coco-Martín MB, Nieto JC. Precision of a commercial Hartmann-Shack aberrometer: limits of total wavefront laser vision correction. Am J Ophthalmol. 2012;154(5):799-807.
5. Liyanage SE, Allan BD. Multiple regression analysis in myopic wavefront laser *in situ* keratomileusis nomogram development. J Cataract Refract Surg. 2012;38(7):1232-9.
6. Deschamps N, Ricaud X, Rabut G, Labbé A, Baudouin C, Denoyer A. The impact of dry eye disease on visual performance while driving. Am J Ophthalmol. 2013;156(1):184-9.
7. Himebaugh NL, Nam J, Bradley A, Liu H, Thibos LN, Begley CG. Scale and spatial distribution of aberrations associated with tear breakup. Optom Vis Sci. 2012;89(11):1590-600.
8. Denoyer A, Rabut G, Baudouin C. Tear film aberration dynamics and vision-related quality of life in patients with dry eye disease. Ophthalmology. 2012;119(9):1811-8.
9. Oliveira CM, Ferreira A, Franco S. Wavefront analysis and Zernike polynomial decomposition for evaluation of corneal optical quality. J Cataract Refract Surg. 2012;38(2):343-56.
10. Saad A, Gatinel D. Evaluation of total and corneal wavefront high order aberrations for the detection of forme fruste keratoconus. Invest Ophthalmol Vis Sci. 2012;53(6):2978-92.
11. Oshika T, Klyce SD, Applegate RA, Howland HC. Changes in corneal wavefront aberrations with aging. Invest Ophthalmol Vis Sci. 1999;40(7):1351-5.
12. Wang L, Dai E, Koch DD, Nathoo A. Optical aberrations of the human anterior cornea. J Cataract Refract Surg. 2003;29(8):1514-21.

13. Dai GM, Mahajan VN. Orthonormal polynomials in wavefront analysis: error analysis. Appl Opt. 2008;47(19):3433-45.

14. Smolek MK, Klyce SD. Goodness-of-prediction of Zernike polynomial fitting to corneal surfaces. J Cataract Refract Surg. 2005;31(12):2350-5.

15. Klyce SD, Karon MD, Smolek MK. Advantages and disadvantages of the Zernike expansion for representing wave aberration of the normal and aberrated eye. J Refract Surg. 2004;20(5): S537-41.

16. Smolek MK, Klyce SD. Zernike polynomial fitting fails to represent all visually significant corneal aberrations. Invest Ophthalmol Vis Sci. 2003;44(11):4676-81.

17. Roorda A. A review of basic wavefront optics. In: Krueger RR, Applegate RA, MacRae SM (Eds). Wavefront Customized Visual Correction; the Quest for Super Vision II. Thorofare, NJ, Slack. 2004;pp.9-18.

18. Maeda N. Clinical applications of wavefront aberrometry: a review. Clin Exp Ophthalmol. 2009;37:118-29.

19. Zhou C, Chai X, Yuan L, He Y, Jin M, Ren Q. Corneal higher-order aberrations after customized aspheric ablation and conventional ablation for myopic correction. Curr Eye Res. 2007;32(5):431-8.

20. Wang Y, Zhao KX, He JC, Jin Y, Zuo T. Ocular higher-order aberrations features analysis after corneal refractive surgery. Chin Med J. 2007;120(4):269-73.

21. Thibos, L, Applegate RA, Schweigerling JT, Webb R. VSIA Standards Taskforce Members, "Standards for Reporting the Optical Aberrations of Eyes," OSA Trends in Optics and Photonics, Vision Science and its Applications, Lakshminarayanan, V (Ed). Optical Society of America, Washington DC. 2000;35:232-44.

CHAPTER **7**

CHAPTER 8

Jorge L Alio, Alfredo Vega Estrada,
Pablo Peña-García

Corneal Aberrometry Changes Following Intracorneal Ring Segment Implantation

INTRODUCTION

The idea of using intracorneal ring segments (ICRS) for the correction of ametropías was developed by JI Barraquer in the early 50's.[1] This technique-based on the thickness law of the same author,[2] states that the addition of tissue in the peripheral cornea or the removal in the center induces a flattening of the cornea. In addition, the postulates of Blavatskaya[2] and Barraquer, states also, that the compensation of the ametropia is directly proportional to the thickness of the segment and inversely proportional to their length.

Although, the physical basis that explains the ICRS performance were known, they were not used in keratoconus patients until the year 2000 when Colin et al.[3] used them for this purpose. They reported a significant flattening of the central cornea and a reduction of the topographic astigmatism, resulting in a more regular shape. They also found a statistically significant reduction in the refractive error, congruent with the topographical effect described. Subsequent studies reported similar results, and evaluated the efficacy and safety of this surgical procedure in keratoconus patients.[4-10] The previous studies showed gain of lines of corrected vision by the patients, in mean terms, however the unpredictability of this treatment has been reported.[11,12] Taking into account the grading system for keratoconus developed by our investigational group, mainly based on the visual status of the patient,[13] it was shown that ICRS implantation can result in a loss of lines of corrected vision in initial grades of keratoconus.[11,12] However, in advanced grades of the illness, results are good enough to consider ICRS implantation as an excellent alternative to prevent, or at least delay, corneal graft.

Regarding the aberrometric changes after ICRS surgery, results are also variable and depend on factors such as, preoperative refractive error, location of the ectasia, and preoperative values of lower and higher order aberrations.

The current nomograms select the number of segments depending on the location of the ectasia. The length and thickness of the segments is determined according to the manifest refraction of the patient. Due to the great variability in refraction, symmetries of the cone and biomechanical behavior of each case, the aberrometric changes are quite variable as mentioned.

The main problem of the refractive compensation in keratoconic eyes is the irregular astigmatism. Therefore, the goal of this surgery is not only to reduce the mean keratometry but also to regularize the corneal shape. The most desirable situation is produced when the steepest meridian is flattened and the flattest meridian is incurved, or when both are flattened but with higher dioptric reduction in the steepest meridian.[14] When this happens, the corneal cylinder diminishes and the root mean square (RMS) of the primary astigmatic aberration (corresponding to the Z(2, 2) and Z(2, –2) Zernike coefficients) is also reduced.

Regarding the high order aberrations (HOA), the spherical-like and coma-like aberrations have been described to have a great influence in the visual function in keratoconic patients.

The ocular spherical aberration is affected by the optics of the cornea and the crystalline lens. Beiko et al[15] reported a mean of +0.27 microns for the spherical aberration induced by the cornea in the normal healthy population. This positive value is compensated by the optics of the crystalline in young patients as reported by Artal et al.[16] However, the ability for the compensation of this aberration declines with age, because the spherical aberration induced by the crystalline lens in older eyes is more positive.

Of course, the changes in the asphericity of the cornea after the implantation of ICRS play an important role in the change of the spherical aberration induced by the cornea and therefore in the ocular spherical aberration. The segments are designed to induce a larger flattening in eyes with higher keratometric values. Normally, the higher the myopia, the higher the flattening and therefore, a more positive spherical aberration is induced.

Therefore, the effect of the segments regarding ocular spherical aberration, depends on the preoperative keratometry, corneal asphericity and age of the patient. Since the spherical aberration has been referred as an important source of visual disturbance, the newest designs of some commercial marks (like the Ferrara segments) have started to consider the corneal asphericity as a parameter to take into account for the selection of the implants.

A mean reduction of the primary coma after the implantation of segments has been reported by most of the authors. The reduction of this aberration, obviously is positive for the visual acuity of the patient, however several studies have investigated this without obtaining a clear conclusion about the preoperative aspects that leads to a reduction of this aberration.[12] Moreover, although in mean terms, the implantation of segments produces a slight reduction of the coma and coma-like aberrations, this reduction could be not statistically significant, at least for all grades.[17]

The type of segments used for the surgery have also influence on the aberrometric changes that happens after the implantation. This issue was studied by our group.[17] Seventeen eyes implanted with INTACS and 20 eyes implanted with Keraring were compared. All the patients included in this study were graded as low-to-moderate keratoconus under the Alió-Shabayeck classification.[18] This classification is mainly based on the aberrometric status of the patients and confers special importance to the coma-like aberrations.

Both implants showed to reduce significantly the spherical equivalent, however, a more limited compensation of the astigmatism was found in the eyes implanted with INTACS. This fact is congruent with a statistically significant higher reduction of the astigmatism RMS in the group of eyes implanted with Keraring. The reason for this different behavior seems to be related with the different length of these two types of segments, shorter in the case of Keraring.

Both implants provided a mean reduction on the primary coma and coma-like aberrations 6 months after the surgery although, this improvement was not statistically significant. In a previous study, it was found statistical significant reduction of the primary coma in those patients with preoperative values coma RMS values higher than 3.0.[19]

Regarding spherical aberration, this study found a significant negativization of the primary spherical aberration in the eyes implanted with INTACS. This effect was not found in the eyes implanted with Kerarring.

Another kind of implant, called Myoring, was also evaluated in a pilot study by our group.[20] The Myoring is a 360° arc length implant, and showed to produce a very powerful flattening of the central cornea, with a mean decrease of 8.00D. Evidently, this behavior has an important impact on the spherical aberration. Although, the sample evaluated was not large (12 eyes), a very significant increment in the corneal primary spherical aberration was noted (p = 0.001) one month after the surgery. However, a significant reduction in the high order aberrations was detected 3 to 6 months after the surgery (p = 0.027).

Finally, the technique used for the implantation of the segments has also been referred as an influent factor on the aberrometric outcomes. In 2009, Alió et al.[21] reported the results of the comparison of mechanical versus femtosecond laser assisted procedures. Although, both techniques achieved similar visual and refractive results, a worse aberrometric correction was found in the case of the manual procedure.

CLINICAL CASES

CASE 1

This case corresponds to a 21 years old female patient with a longstanding history of keratoconus who wear contact lenses during the last seven years. During the last six months she referred intolerance to contact lens on her right eye and she notice that her visual acuity has decrease over the last few months.

Ophthalmological Evaluation

Uncorrected visual acuity (UCVA)
Right eye (RE): 0.050.
Left eye (LE): 0.200.

Corrected visual acuity (CDVA)
Right eye (RE): 0.800.
Left eye (LE): 1.00.

Refraction
RE: Sph –3.00 cyl –3.00@140°.
LE: Sph –2.50 cyl –2.00@30.

Biomicroscopy
RE: Transparent cornea, peripheral nerve thickening.
LE: Unremarkable.

Fundus evaluation
Unremarkable.

Corneal pachymetry
RE: 458 microns.
LE: 480 microns.

Preoperative Corneal Topography (Fig. 1)

RE: Central oval pattern with flattest keratometry (K1): 47.82 D and steepest keratometry (K2): 52.03D.
LE: Normal.

Preoperative Corneal Aberrometry (Fig. 2)

RE
RMS total: 9.50 microns.
RMS coma: 2.41 microns.
RMS spherical aberration: 1.66 microns.
Surgical planning: We decided to perform an implantation of two intracorneal ring segments (ICRS) on the right eye following the guidelines of the manufacturer´s nomogram.

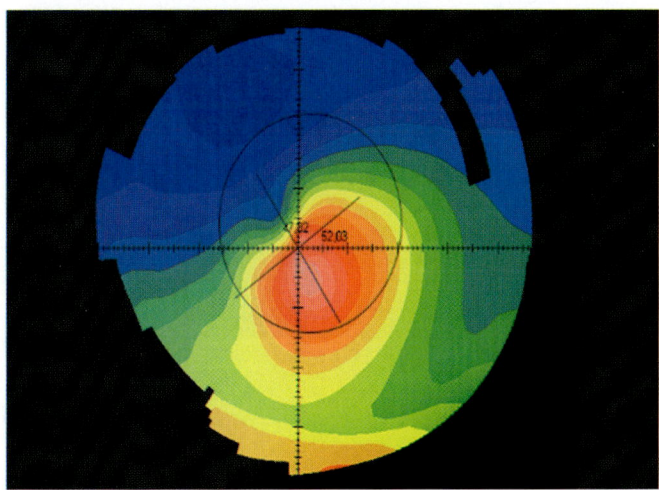

Fig. 1: Keratokonus preoperative

Postoperative Evaluation

Ophthalmological evaluation six months after the procedure showed the following findings:

UCVA
Right eye (RE): 0.300.
Spectacle CDVA (RE): 0.840.
Contact lens CDVA (RE): 1.000.
Refraction: Sph –1.50 cyl –2.50@140°.

Postoperative Corneal Topography and Aberrometry (Figs 3 and 4)

K1: 46.74D.
K2: 51.39D.
RMS total aberrations: 7.53 microns.
RMS coma aberration: 1.24 microns.

Summary

This case correspond to a mild keratoconus case taking into account the level of anterior corneal aberrations and the degree of visual limitation. After implantation of two ICRS around the central zone of the cornea which correspond to the focal steepening in the corneal topography, we found a central flattening of the area that leads to a reduction in the spherical equivalent of the patient. We also observed an important reduction of more than 1 micron in the root mean square of the coma aberration that certainly will increase the optical quality of the patient.

CHAPTER **8**

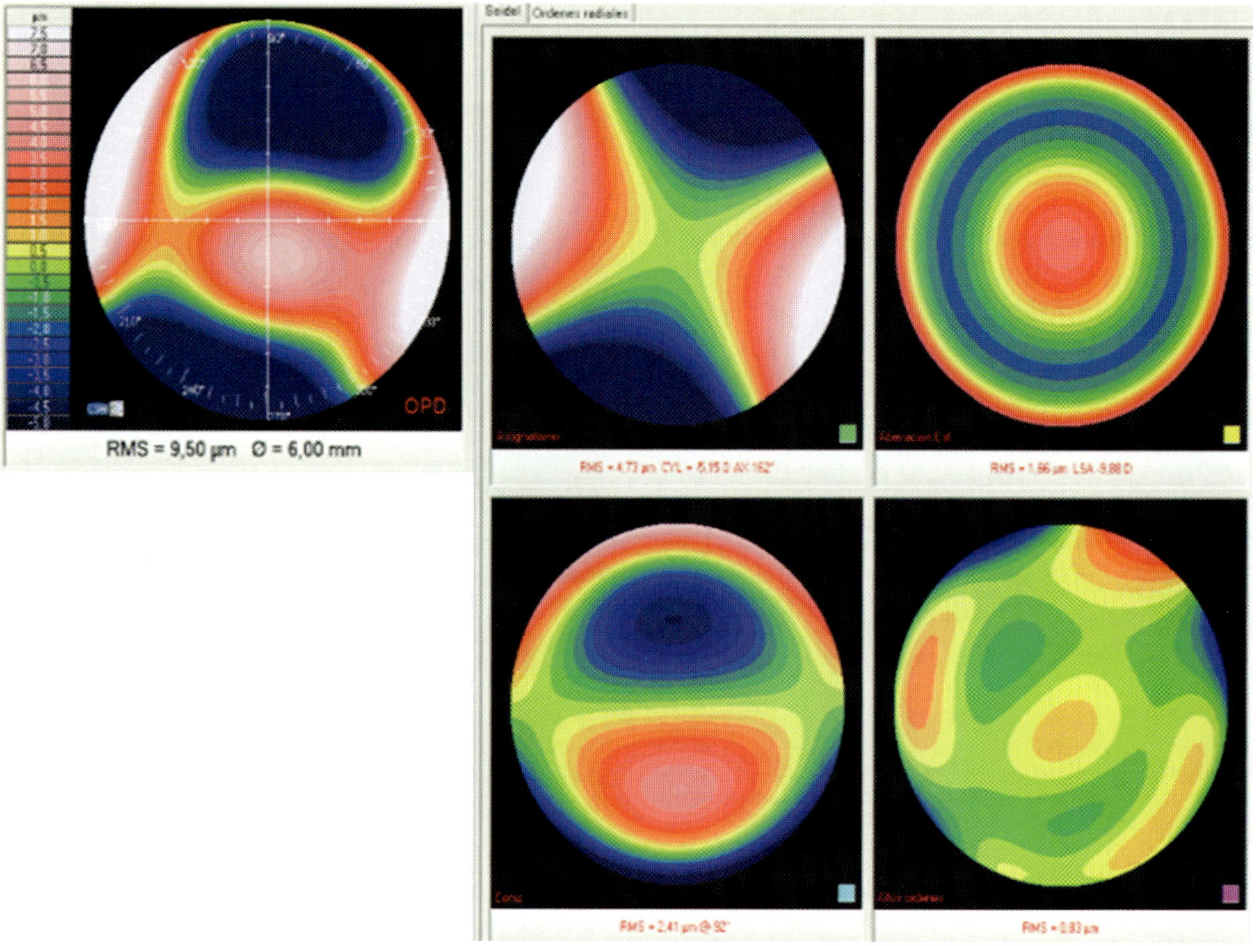

RMS = 9,50 µm   Ø = 6,00 mm

OPD

Soidel | Ordenes radiales |

RMS = 4,73 µm CYL = -5,15 D AX 162°

RMS = 1,66 µm LSA -9,88 D

RMS = 2,41 µm @ 92°

RMS = 0,93 µm

Fig. 2: Preoperative

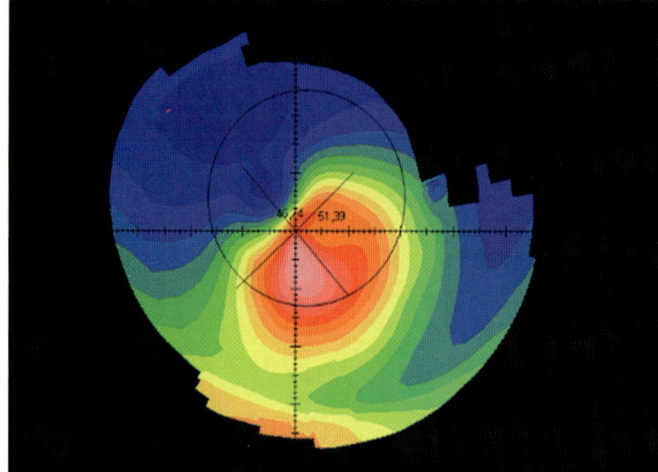

Fig. 3: Postoperative

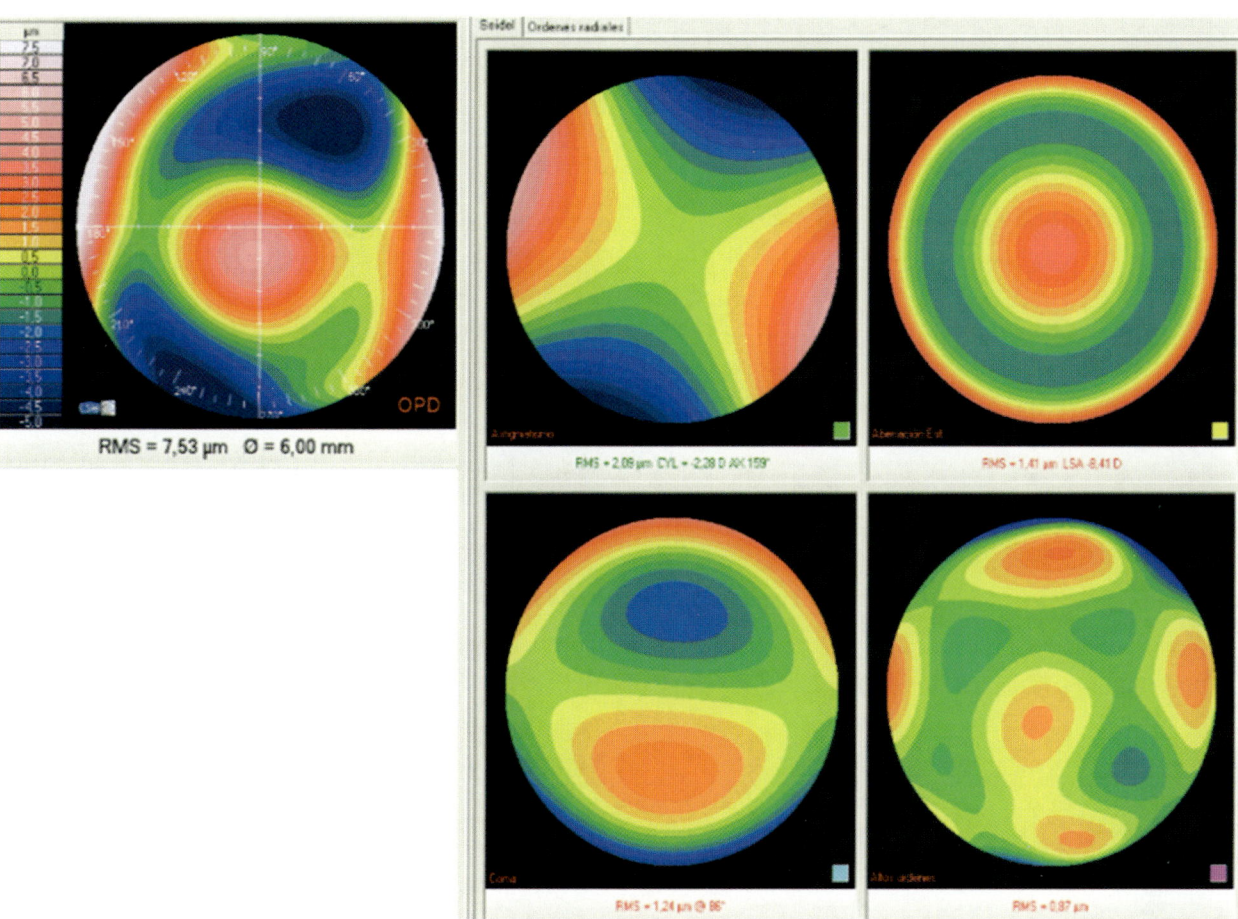

Fig. 4: Postoperative

CASE 2

This case corresponds to a 26 years old female patient with a longstanding history of keratoconus who has a poor motivation to contact lens wearing.

Ophthalmological Evaluation

UCVA
RE: 0.100.
LE: 0.100.

CDVA
RE: 0.600.
LE: 0.800.

Refraction
RE: Sph +1.50 cyl –4.25@80°.
LE: Sph cyl –2.00@110.

Biomicroscopy
RE: Corneal thinning, Fleischer ring.
LE: Unremarkable.

Fundus evaluation
Unremarkable.

Corneal pachymetry
RE: 419 microns.
LE: 472 microns.

Preoperative Corneal Topography (Fig. 5)

RE: Inferior steepening and asymmetric bowtie pattern.
K1: 52.18D.
K2: 58.37D.

Preoperative Corneal Aberrometry (Fig. 6)

RE
RMS total: 40.00 microns.
RMS coma: 3.70 microns.
RMS spherical aberration: –0.58 microns.
Surgical planning: We decided to perform an implantation of one ICRS inferiorly on the right eye as suggested by the guidelines of the manufacturer´s nomogram.

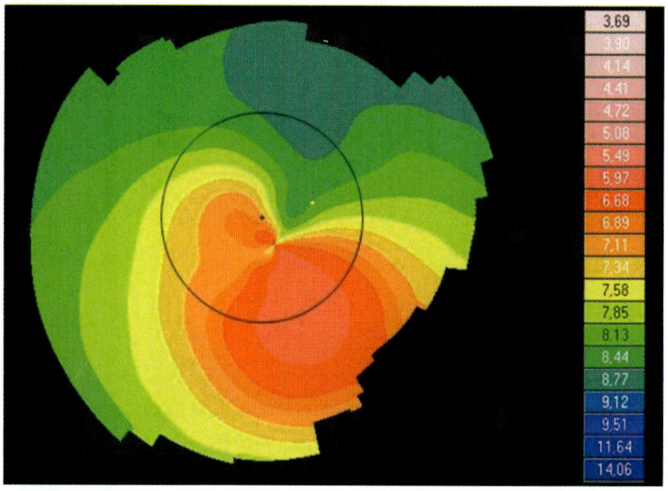

Fig. 5: Keratokonus preoperative

Postoperative Evaluation

Ophthalmological evaluation six months after the procedure showed the following findings:

UCVA
Right eye (RE): 0.500.
CDVA (RE): 0.800.

Refraction
Sph 0.00 cyl –2.50@110°.

Postoperative Corneal Topography and Aberrometry (Figs 7 and 8)

K1: 51.75D.
K2: 55.13D.
RMS total aberrations: 16.06 micorns.
RMS coma aberration: 1.36 microns.

Summary

This case corresponds to a moderate keratoconus case taking into account the level of anterior corneal aberrations and the degree of visual limitation. Inferiorly implantation of one ICRS leads to a "push up" of the inferior steepening towards the center of the cornea which induces a more regular anterior corneal surface with the consequent reduction of more than 2 microns in the asymmetric (coma) aberration.

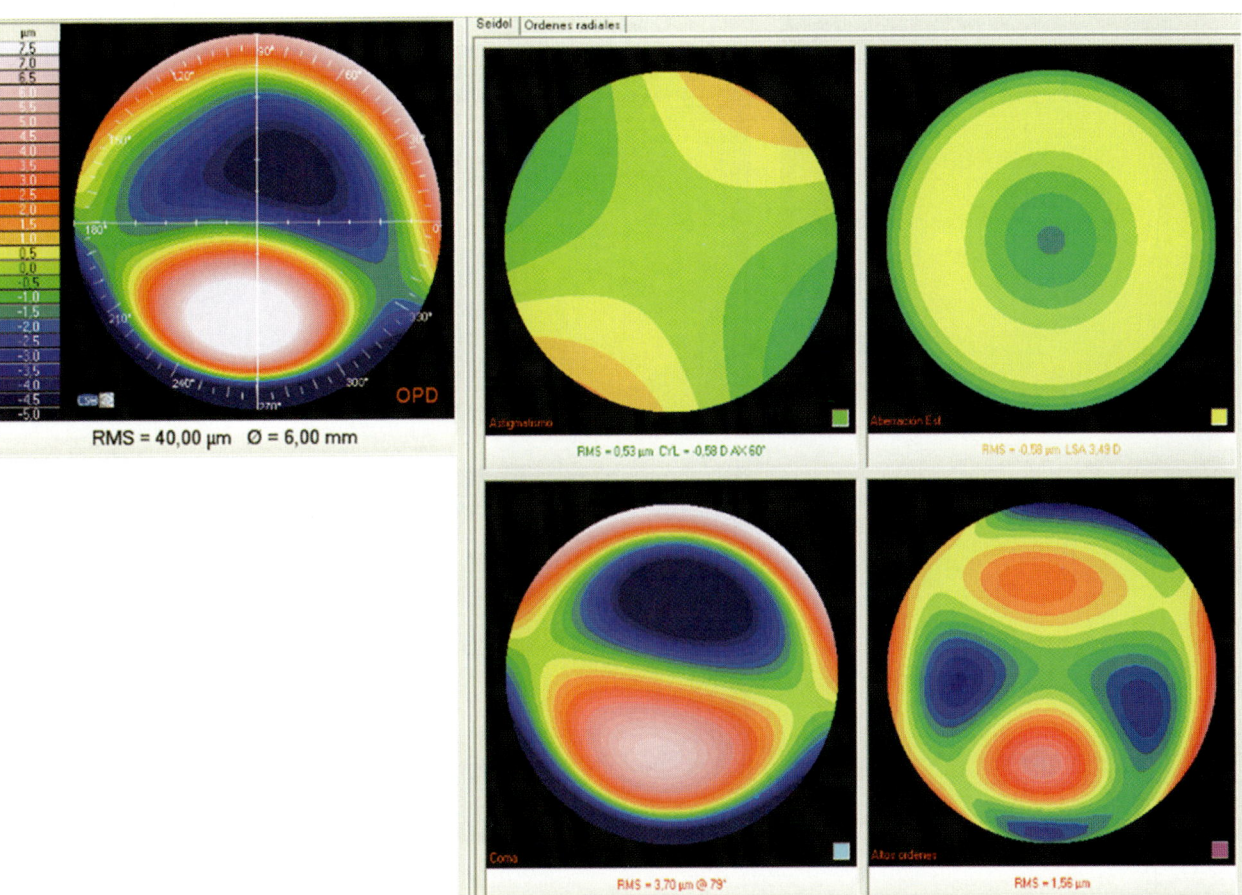

Fig. 6: Preoperative

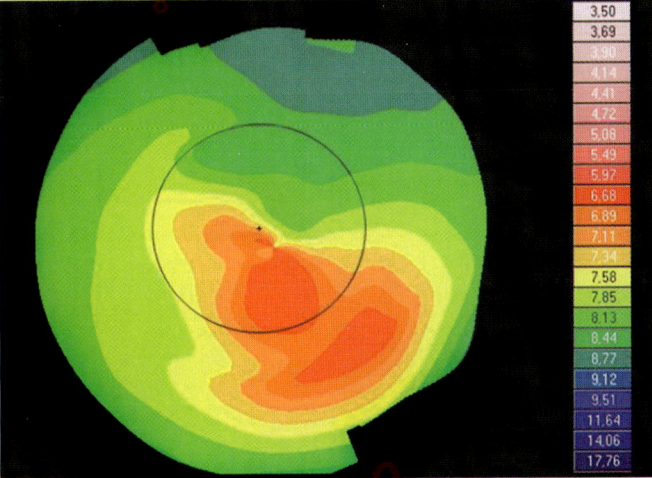

Fig. 7: Postoperative

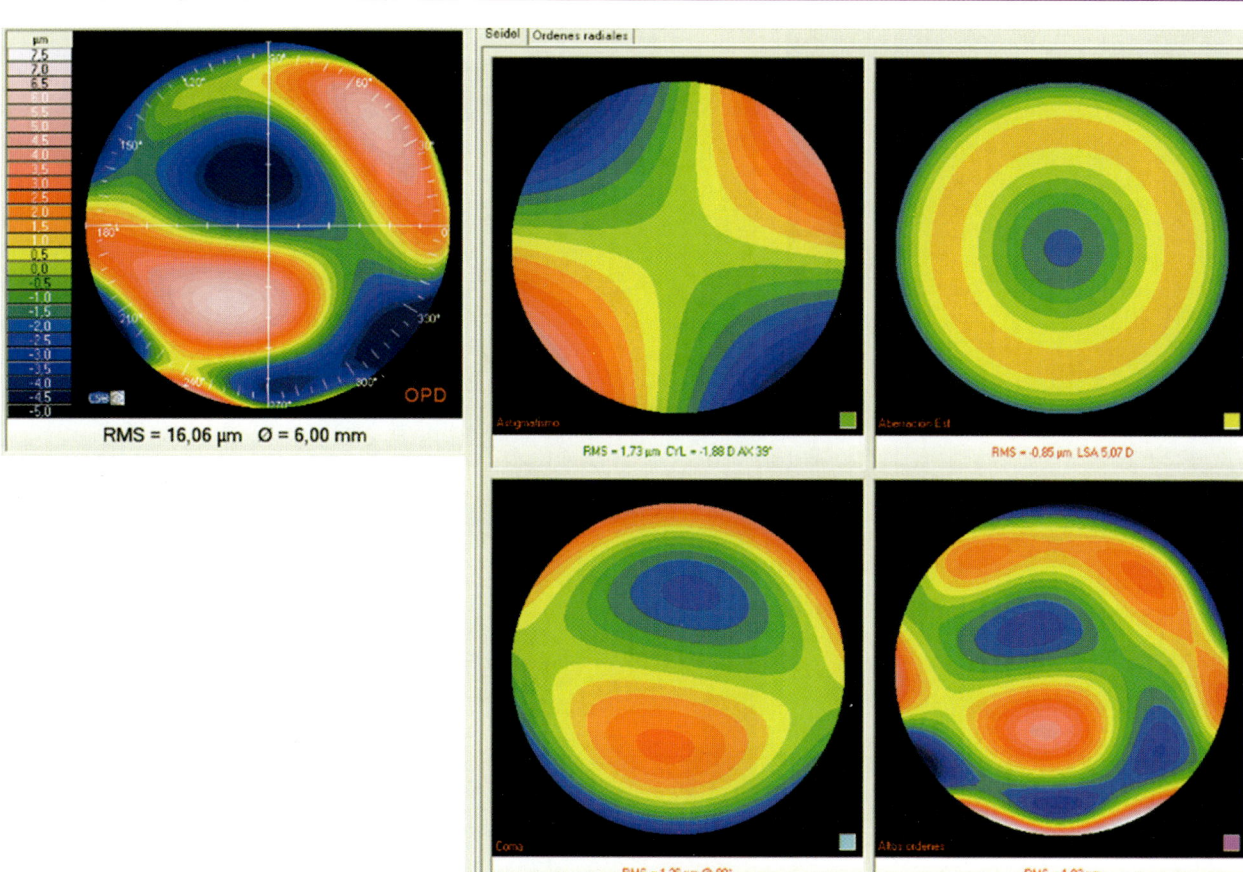

Fig. 8: Postoperative

CASE 3

The last case corresponds to a 25 years old male patient with a longstanding history of keratoconus who underwent a penetrating keratoplasty procedure 3 years ago on the right eye. He is referred to our center to evaluate the possibility of performing a deep anterior lamellar keratoplasty (DALK) on the left eye.

Ophthalmological Evaluation

UCVA
RE: 0.500.
LE: Counting fingers at 3 meters.

CDVA
RE: 0.900.
LE: 0.320.

Refraction
RE: Sph –1.00 cyl –2.00@10°.
LE: Sph –7.50 cyl –4.00@60.

Biomicroscopy
RE: Transparent corneal graft.
LE: Central corneal thinning, Vogt striae, transparent cornea without central leucoma.

Fundus evaluation
Unremarkable.

Corneal pachymetry
RE: 570 microns.
LE: 361 microns.

Preoperative Corneal Topography (Fig. 9)

LE: Central oval pattern with a severe central steepening.
K1: 53.67D.
K2: 60.29D.

Preoperative Corneal Aberrometry (Fig. 10)

LE
• **RMS total:** 29.01 microns.
• **RMS coma:** 4.94 microns.
• **RMS spherical aberration:** 0.91 microns.
Surgical planning: Even though the visual acuity and the prognosis of this case was very poor we discuss the different therapeutic alternative with the patient and decided to offer him ICRS implantation leaving the DALK procedure for the future in case that ICRS implantation failed. We decided to perform an implantation of two ICRS following the guidelines of the manufacturer's nomogram.

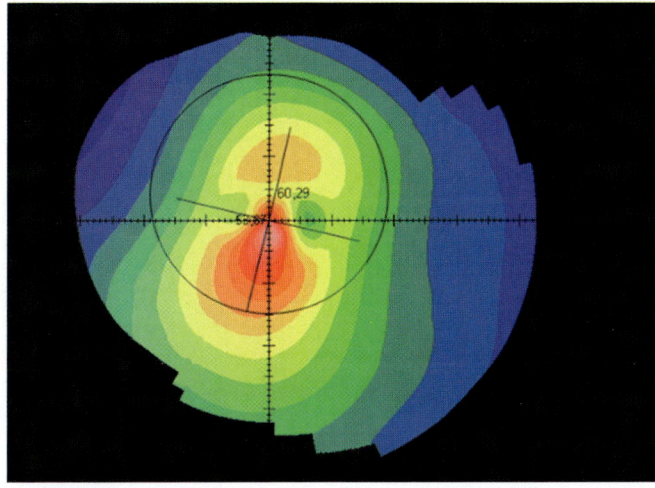

Fig. 9: Keratokonus preoperative

Postoperative Evaluation

Ophthalmological evaluation six months after the procedure showed the following findings:

UCVA
LE: 0.300.

Spectacle CDVA
LE: 0.500.

Contact lens CDVA
LE: 0.700.

Refraction
Sph –3.00 cyl –2.25@140°.

Postoperative Corneal Topography and Aberrometry (Figs 11 and 12)

K1: 53.85D.
K2: 56.62D.
RMS total aberrations: 7.46.
RMS coma aberration: 1.69 microns.

Summary

This case correspond to a severe keratoconus case taking into account the level of anterior corneal aberrations and the degree of visual limitation. We found that after ICRS implantation there is a flattening of the central cornea and a major reduction of the coma aberration that improves the visual function and the refraction of the patient. The modeling effect of the corneal stroma observed after implantation of the segments allow us in this case not just to achieved an important reduction of the anterior corneal aberrations but to delay or even avoid a keratoplasty procedure in a young patient.

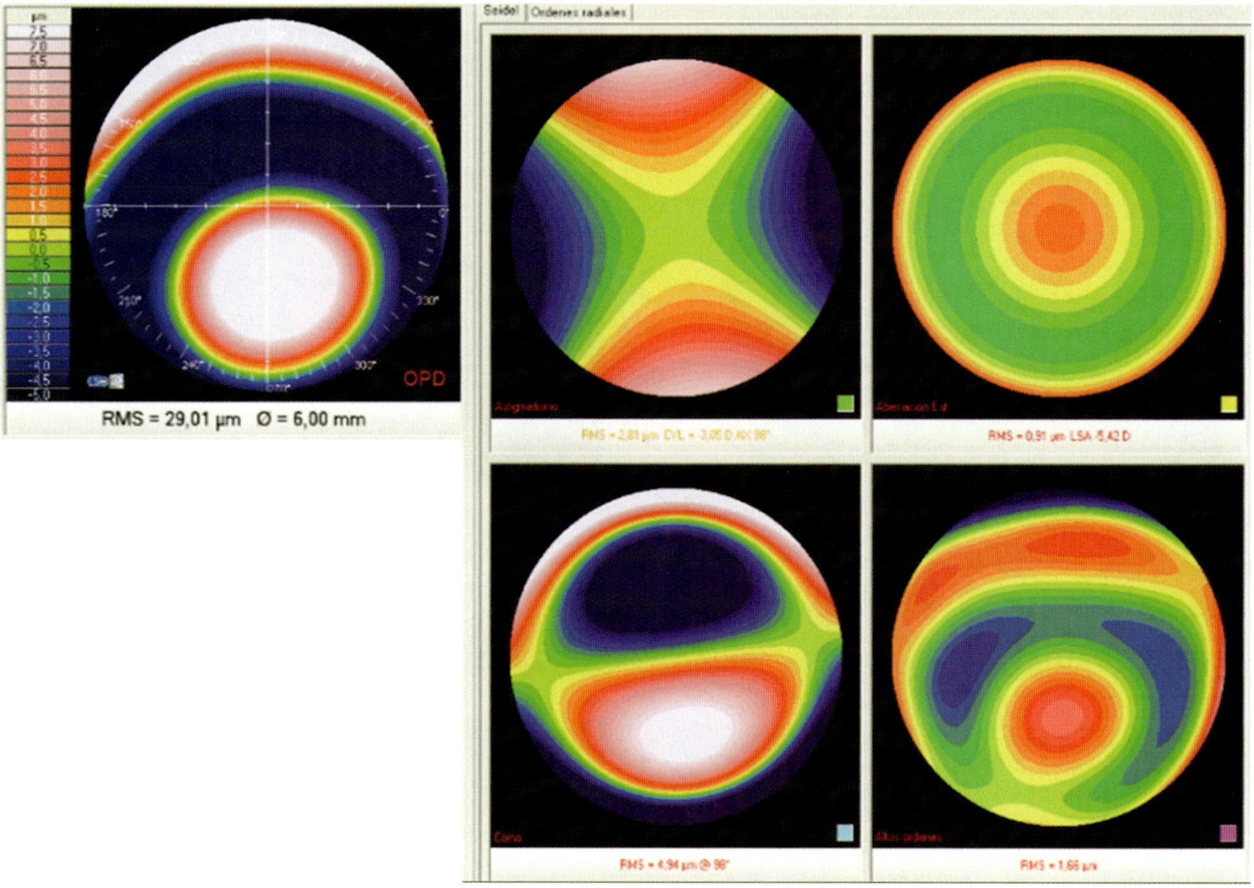

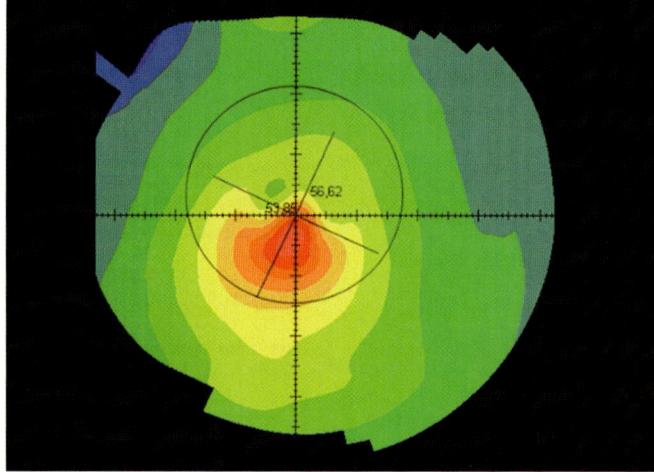

RMS = 29,01 µm   Ø = 6,00 mm

Fig. 10: Preoperative

Fig. 11: Postoperative

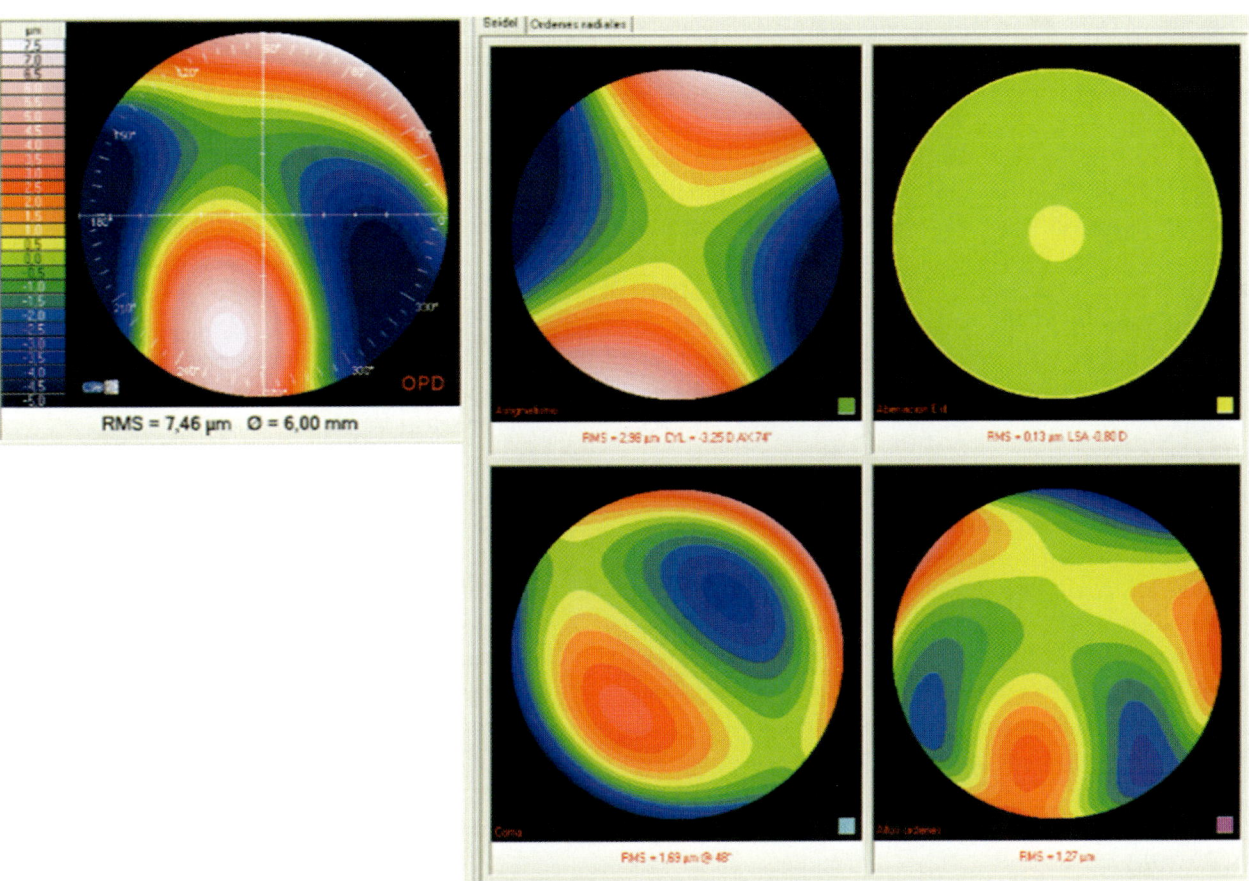

Fig. 12: Postoperative

REFERENCES

1. Barraquer JI. Queratoplastia refractiva, estudios e informaciones oftalmológicas. 1949;2:10-30.

2. Barraquer JI. Cirugía Refractiva de la Córnea. Instituto Barraquer de América- Bogotá, Tomo I, 1989.

3. Colin J, Cochener B, Savary G, Malet F. Correcting keratoconus with intracorneal rings. J Cataract Refract Surg. 2000;26: 1117-22.

4. Alió JL, Salem TF, Artola A, Osman AA. Intracorneal rings to correct corneal ectasia after laser *in situ* keratomileusis. J Cataract Refract Surg. 2002;28:1568-74.

5. Siganos CS, Kymionis GD, Kartakis N, Theodorakis MA, Astyrakakis N, Pallikaris IG. Management of keratoconus with Intacs. Am J Ophthalmol. 2003;135:64-70.

6. Ruckhofer J, Stoiber J, Twa MD, Grabner G. Correction of astigmatism with short arc-length intrastromal corneal ring segments; preliminary results. Ophthalmology. 2003;110: 516-24.

7. Kymionis GD, Siganos CS, Kounis G, Astyrakakis N, Kalyvianaki MI, Pallikaris IG. Management of post-LASIK corneal ectasia with Intacs inserts; one-year results. Arch Ophthalmol. 2003;121:322-6.

8. Barbara A, Shehadeh-Masha'our R, Zvi R, Garzozi HJ. Management of pellucid marginal degeneration with intracorneal ring segments. J Refract Surg. 2005;21:296-8.

9. Alió JL, Shabayek MH, Artola A. Intracorneal ring segments for keratoconus correction: long-term follow-up. J Cataract Refract Surg. 2006;32:978-85.

10. Shabayek MH, Alió JL. Intrastromal corneal ring segment implantation by femtosecond laser for keratoconus correction. Ophthalmology. 2007;114:1643-52.

11. Vega-Estrada A, Alio JL, Brenner LF, Javaloy J, Plaza Puche AB, Barraquer RI, Teus MA, Murta J, Henriques J, Uceda-

CHAPTER 8

Montanes A. Outcome analysis of intracorneal ring segments for the treatment of keratoconus based on visual, refractive, and aberrometric impairment. Am J Ophthalmol. 2013;155(3): 575-84.

12. Peña-García P, Vega-Estrada A, Barraquer RI, Burguera-Giménez N, Alio JL. Intracorneal ring segment in keratoconus: a model to predict visual changes induced by the surgery. Invest Ophthalmol Vis Sci. 2012;53(13):8447-57.

13. Alió JL, Piñero DP, Alesón A, Teus MA, Barraquer RI, Murta J, Maldonado MJ, Castro de Luna G, Gutiérrez R, Villa C, Uceda-Montanes A. Keratoconus-integrated characterization considering anterior corneal aberrations, internal astigmatism, and corneal biomechanics. J Cataract Refract Surg. 2011;37(3):552-68.

14. Albertazzi R. Tratamiento del queratocono con segmentos intracorneales. Editor: Albertazzi R. Queratocono: pautas para su diagnostico y tratamiento. Buenos Aires. Ediciones Científicas Argentinas para la Keratoconus Society. 2010:205-67.

15. Beiko GH, Haigis W, Steinmueller A. Distribution of corneal spherical aberration in a comprehensive ophthalmology practice and whether keratometry can predict aberration values. J Cataract Refract Surg. 2007;33(5):848-58.

16. Artal P, Berrio E, Guirao A, Piers P. Contribution of the cornea and internal surfaces to the change of ocular aberrations with age. J Opt Soc Am A Opt Image Sci Vis. 2002;19(1):137-43.

17. Piñero DP, Alió JL, El Kady B, Pascual I. Corneal aberrometric and refractive performance of 2 intrastromal corneal ring segment models in early and moderate ectatic disease. J Cataract Refract Surg. 2010;36(1):102-9.

18. Alió JL, Shabayek MH. Corneal higher order aberrations: a method to grade keratoconus. J Refract Surg. 2006;22(6): 539-45.

19. Shabayek MH, Alió JL. Intrastromal corneal ring segment implantation by femtosecond laser for keratoconus correction. Ophthalmology. 2007;114:1643-52.

20. Alio JL, Piñero DP, Daxer A. Clinical outcomes after complete ring implantation in corneal ectasia using the femtosecond technology: a pilot study. Ophthalmology. 2011;118(7): 1282-90.

21. Piñero DP, Alio JL, El Kady B, Coskunseven E, Morbelli H, Uceda-Montanes A, Maldonado MJ, Cuevas D, Pascual I. Refractive and aberrometric outcomes of intracorneal ring segments for keratoconus: mechanical versus femtosecond-assisted procedures. Ophthalmology. 2009;116(9):1675-87.

3
SECTION

CHAPTER 9

Monocular Diplopia

EXAMPLE OF TOPO-GUIDED ABLATION

Here you will find some examples of post-LASIK significant visual complains such as monocular diplopia. The irregular astigmatism was treated with CIPTA Software (topo-guided ablation): symptoms were reduced and UCVA improved.

Case 1

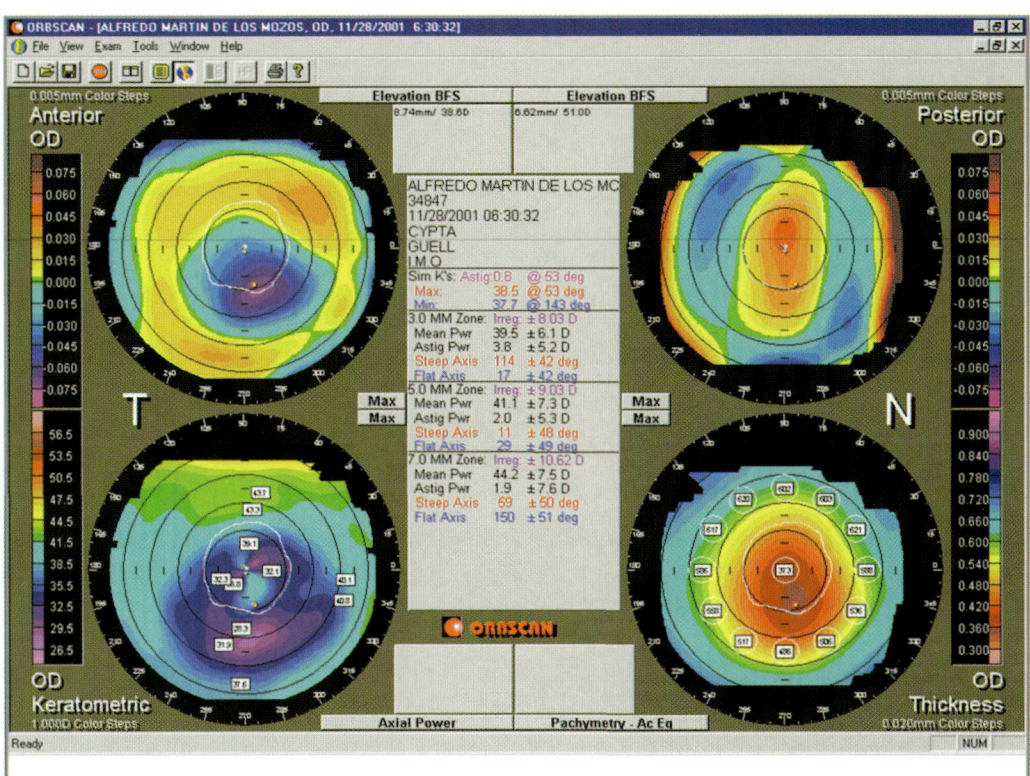

50°-1.00 + 2.00 VA 0.2 + "ghost image"

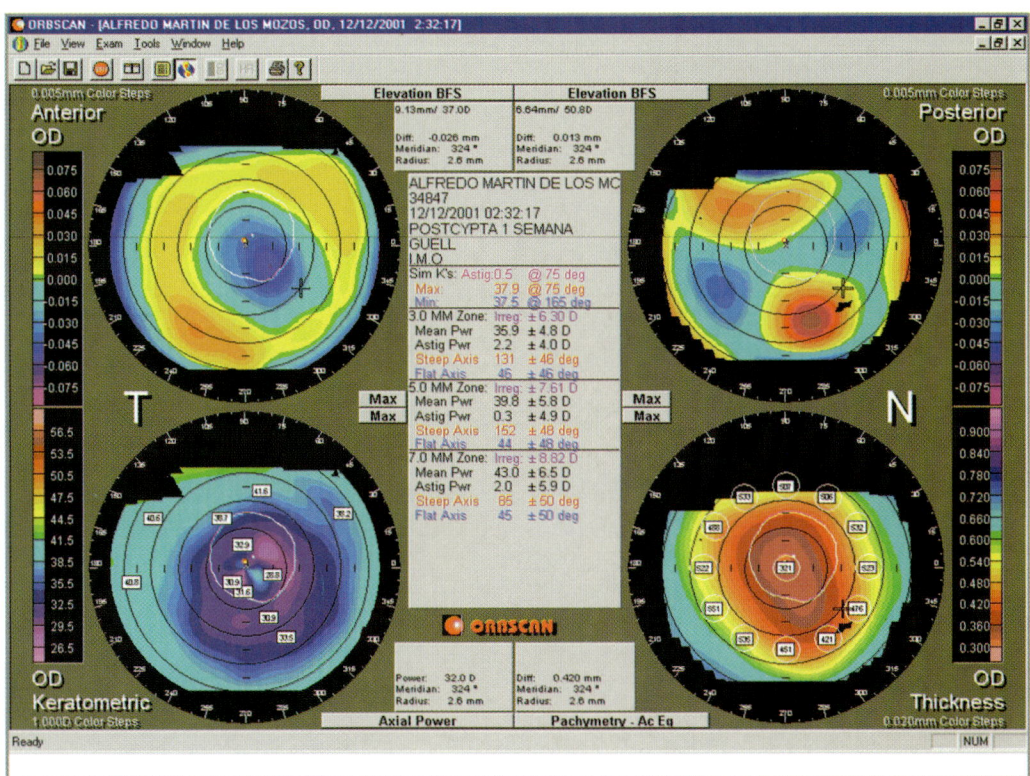

10°-2.00 + 1.50 VA 0.63

Case 2

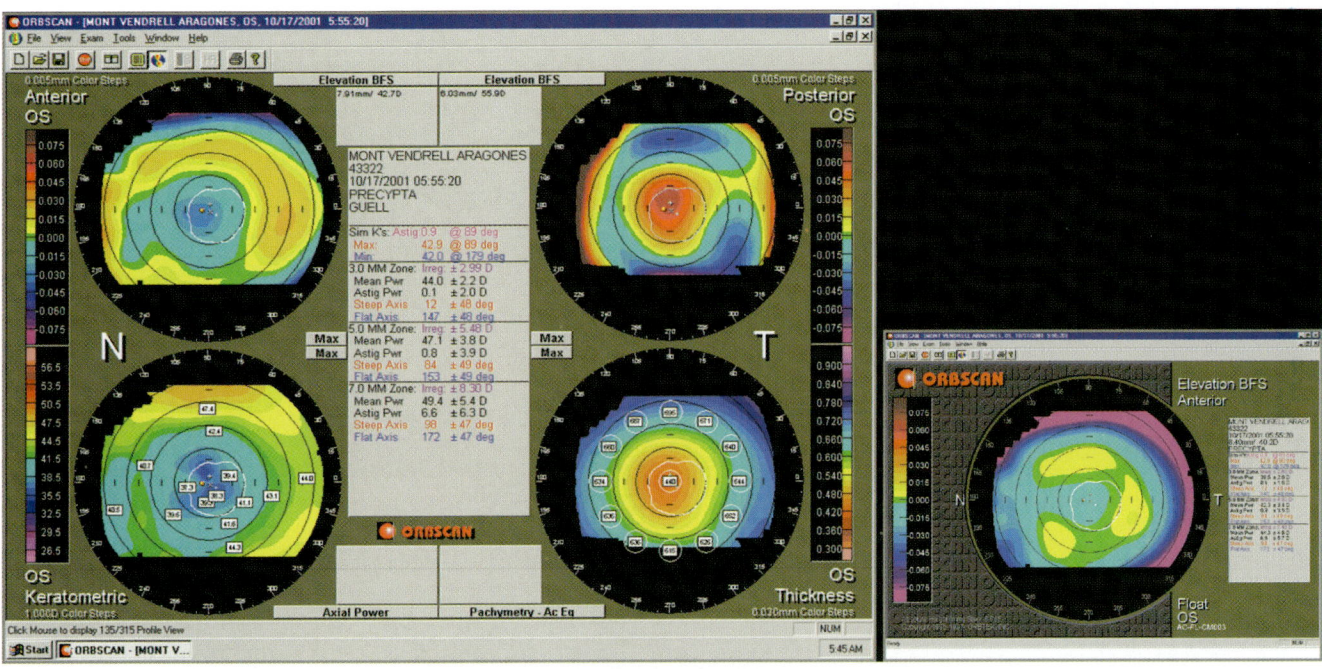

UCVA 0.25 (120°-1.00 + 2.00) 0.4 + monocular diplopia

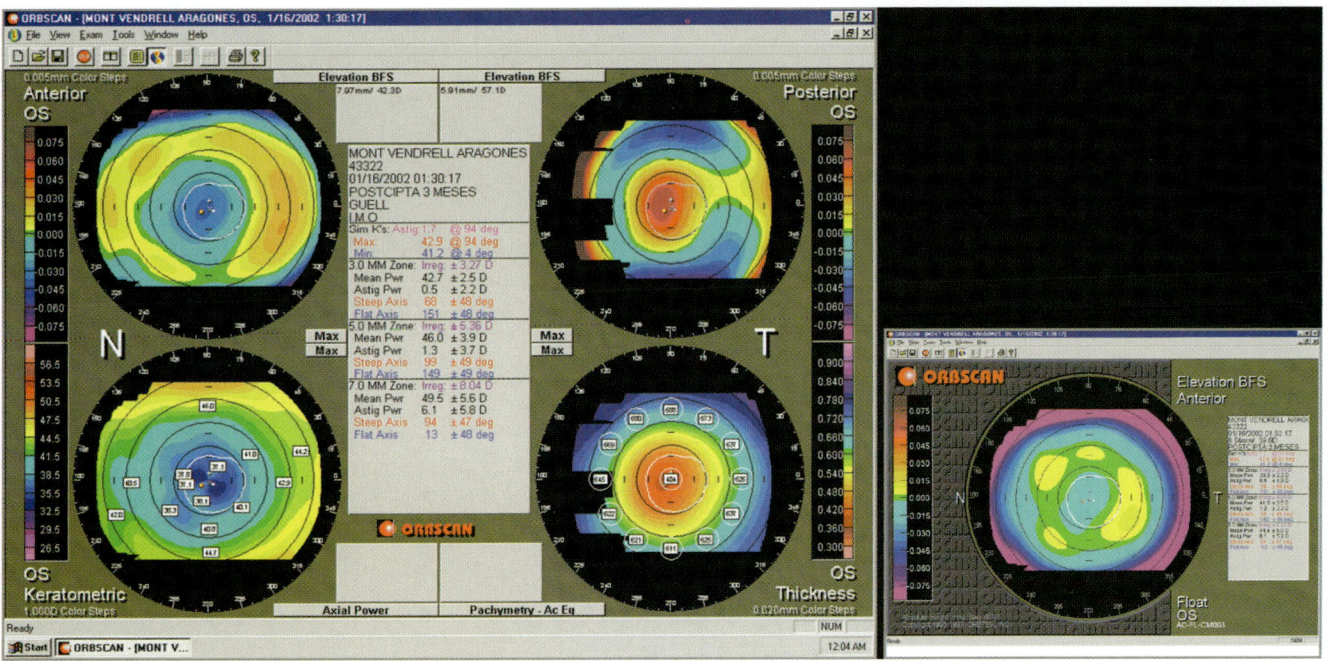

UCVA 0.4 – (120°-0.50 + 1.50) 0.6 + no monocular diplopia

Case 3

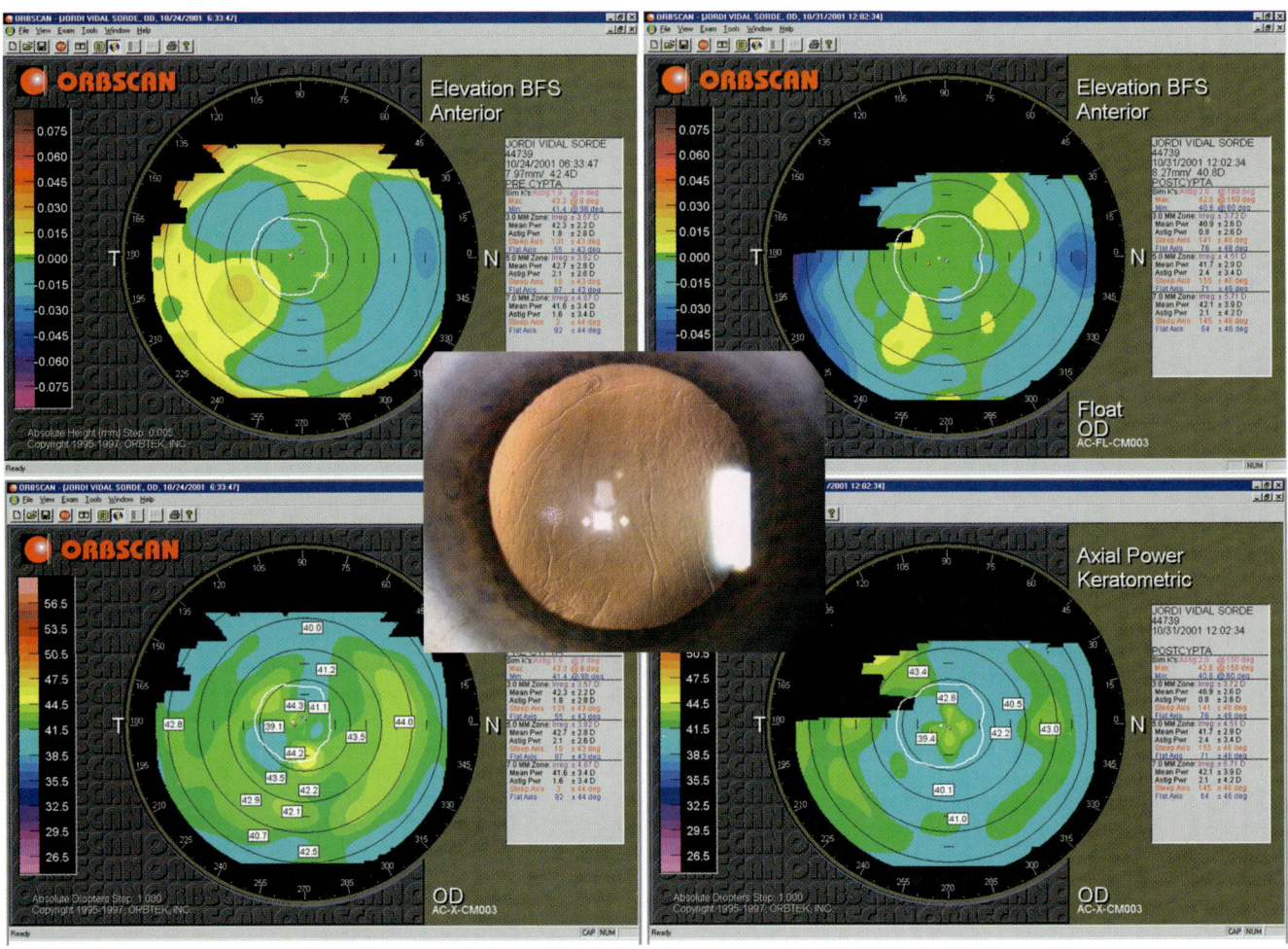

UCVA 0.2 (70°-3.00 + 2.25) 0.5 – pinhole 0.8 – monocular diplopia   UCVA 0.6 (55°-0.75 + 0.50) 0.8 – no monocular diplopia

Case 4

UCVA 0.2- (25°-4.00 + 0.50) 0.3-blurred   **UCVA 0.4 (110°-2.00 + 1.25) 0.6-clear**

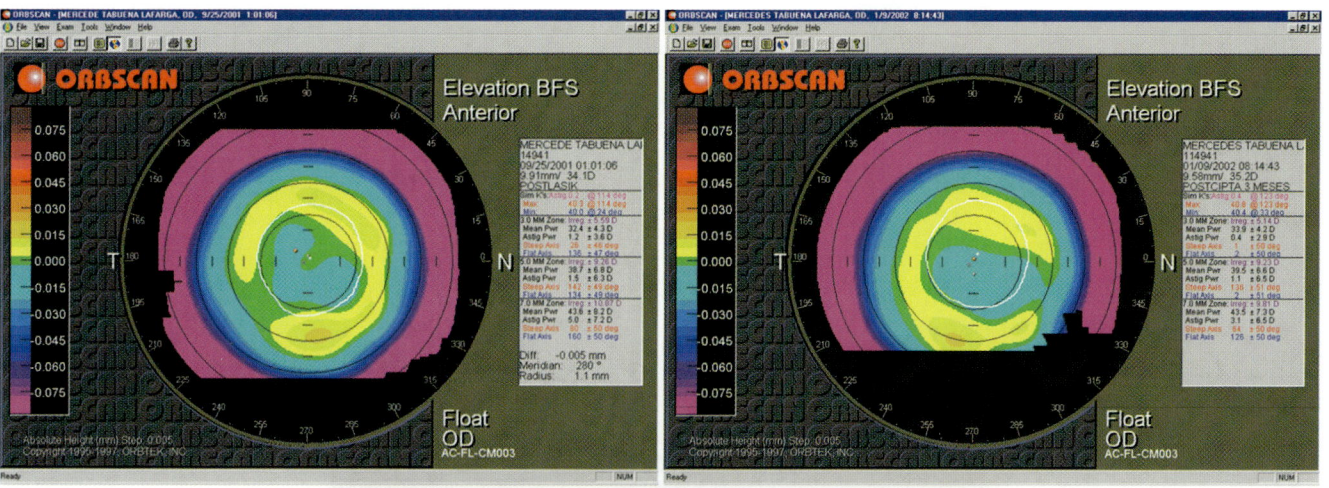

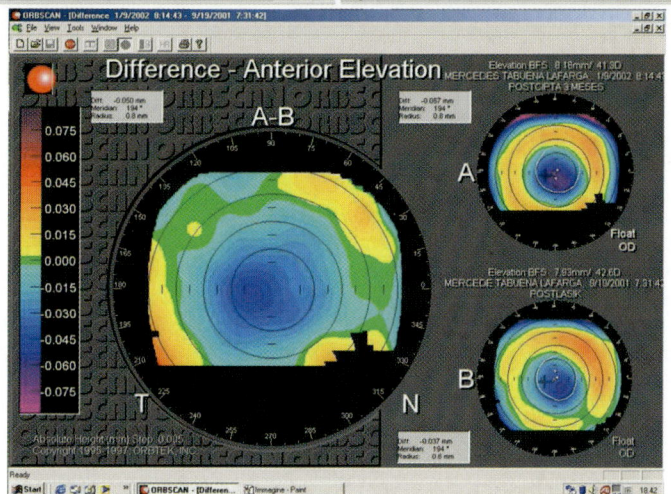

CHAPTER 10

Peter S Hersh, Yinfei Xu, David S Chu

Wavefront Analysis and Scheimpflug Imagery in Diagnosis of Anterior Lenticonus

Abstract

We present the case of an Alport syndrome patient whose anterior lenticonus was detected by wavefront analysis and Scheimpflug imaging technology. Patient's lenticular abnormalities were too subtle to be detected by the initial slit-lamp examination. However, normal corneal topography and elevation maps with high total eye aberrations pointed to internal optics as the source of aberrations. More specifically, predominant negative spherical aberrations suggested anterior lenticonus, a diagnosis further confirmed by Scheimpflug images showing central bulging of the anterior lens surface. Following diagnosis, patient underwent successful phacoemulsification and intraocular lens (IOL) implantation. We recommend wavefront analysis and Scheimpflug imaging technology as effective tools in the detection of lens disorders, especially those that are too subtle to be observed by other examination methods.

INTRODUCTION

Anterior lenticonus (AL) is a rare condition in which a portion of the crystalline lens capsule and underlying cortex bulge anteriorly. The conical protrusion results from a genetic defect in synthesis of type IV collagen, a major component of the lenticular basement membrane.[1] AL develops progressively and bilaterally, possibly manifesting as severe myopia and lenticular irregular astigmatism.[2] Although sometimes isolated, AL may also present as a pathognomonic feature of Alport syndrome, a hereditary nephritis accompanied by sensorineural hearing loss as well as other ocular abnormalities.[3] AL occurs in approximately 25% of patients with X-linked Alport syndrome.[4] Posterior lenticonus is not usually associated with a systematic disease.[5]

Several literatures have reported success in treatment of AL. Liu et al[5] recommend phacoemulsification with foldable IOL implantation as a safe and efficient procedure. However, the disorder must be diagnosed before it can be treated, a process that may sometimes prove difficult. Because the change in lens contour is often very subtle, AL can remain undetected throughout ocular examinations. New imaging technology, such as wavefront sensing and Schiempflug imaging, can help in the early diagnosis of such optical disorders.

To demonstrate these technologies as important tools in diagnosing anterior lenticonus and other optical disorders, we present an Alport syndrome patient whose subtle lenticular abnormalities were first detected by wavefront analysis and then confirmed by Scheimpflug quantitative imaging.

CASE REPORT AND METHODS

A 44-year-old male with Alport syndrome was referred to our clinic to be considered for refractive surgery. His chief complaint was a progressive reduction of vision in both eyes and he sought the procedure in hopes of improving his vision. Ocular symptoms were managed by wearing prescription glasses but best corrected visual acuity (BCVA) remained unsatisfactory. Past ocular histories were otherwise unremarkable. Patient had a history of renal failure and kidney transplant twenty-one years previously. His medications included prednisone, cyclosporine, magox, soriatune, nexium, norvasc, atorvastatin calcium, warfarin sodium, colchicines, niferex, atenolol, doxercalciferol, fenofibrate, folic acid, duloxetine hydrochloride, foltx, allopurinol, and digoxin.

On examination, uncorrected visual acuity was $20/50^{-1}$ OD and 20/70 OS. BCVA and subjective manifest refraction was $20/30^{-1}$ OD with –6.25 –1.00 × 155 and $20/40^{-2}$ OS with –7.25 –2.50 × 170. Slit-lamp biomicroscopy revealed a clear and compact cornea with normal intraocular pressure and fundi. No significant cataract or other obvious anomalies of the lens and anterior segment were observed.

Corneal topographic and elevation maps were normal as computed by the OCULUS Pentacam software (OCULUS, Lynnwood WA, USA). Sagittal curvature and elevation maps of the patient's cornea front are shown in **Figure 1**.

Wavefront analysis was performed with the Alcon LADARWave aberrometer (Alcon Labs, Fort Worth, Texas, USA). The device utilizes Hartmann-Shack principles to detect, measure, and display higher order aberrations of the eye. Total-eye wavefront analysis revealed high negative spherical aberration in both eyes with RMS values of –1.08 μm and –1.43 μm for right and left eyes, respectively. Preoperative wavefront maps with Zernike modes and aberration values are shown in **Figures 2A to C**. Given normal corneal maps and abnormal total-eye wavefront analysis, the internal optics of the eye, thus, was likely the main source of vision deficits. More specifically, previous literature indicated

that predominant spherical aberrations were suggestive of anterior lenticonus (AL).[6]

The OCULUS Pentacam is also able to define the anterior curvature of the lens. Rotating Scheimpflug imaging with the Pentacam captures twenty-five image slices from the anterior surface of the cornea to the posterior surface of the lens.[5] These images detailed the contour of the protrusion in our patient's dilated lens over a 360-degree circle. Scheimpflug images in **Figures 3A to C** display the anterior lenticonus in our patient against that of a normal lens.

To characterize this Scheimpflug image of lenticonus and compare it to the normal population, measurements were taken from the apex of the bulge to a 4 mm chord length for fifteen refractive surgery candidates with normal lenses. Variability was minimized by including only dilated lenses and candidates within 6 years of age from our patient. Measurements yielded a 400 μm protrusion in the lenticonus eye reported herein compared to a mean of 256.7 μm with 27.2 μm standard deviation for those without lenticular abnormalities (**Figs 3A to C**).

Since ocular symptoms were most severe in the left eye, cataract extraction and IOL implantation were selected to be performed first on the left eye. Following lens removal through phacoemulsification, an ACRYSOF® IOL, manufactured by Alcon Labs, Fort Worth, Texas, was inserted into the eye.

DISCUSSION

This case highlights the role of wavefront analysis and Scheimpflug imaging technology in detecting lenticular

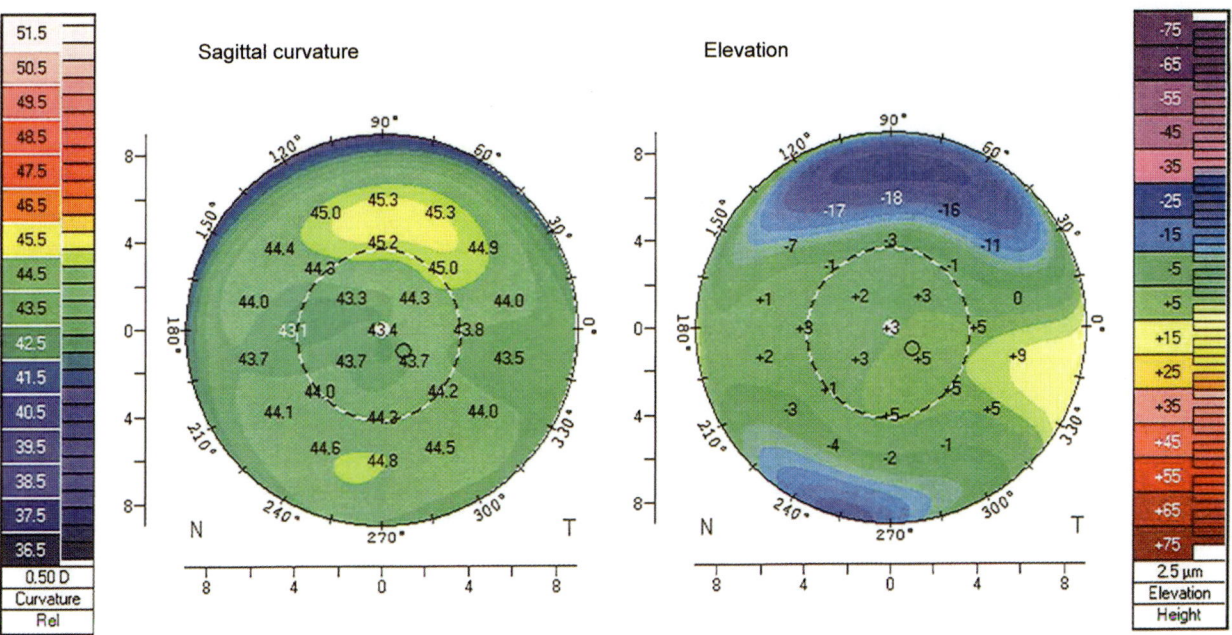

Fig. 1: Normal left eye corneal front topographic maps of sagittal curvature and elevation

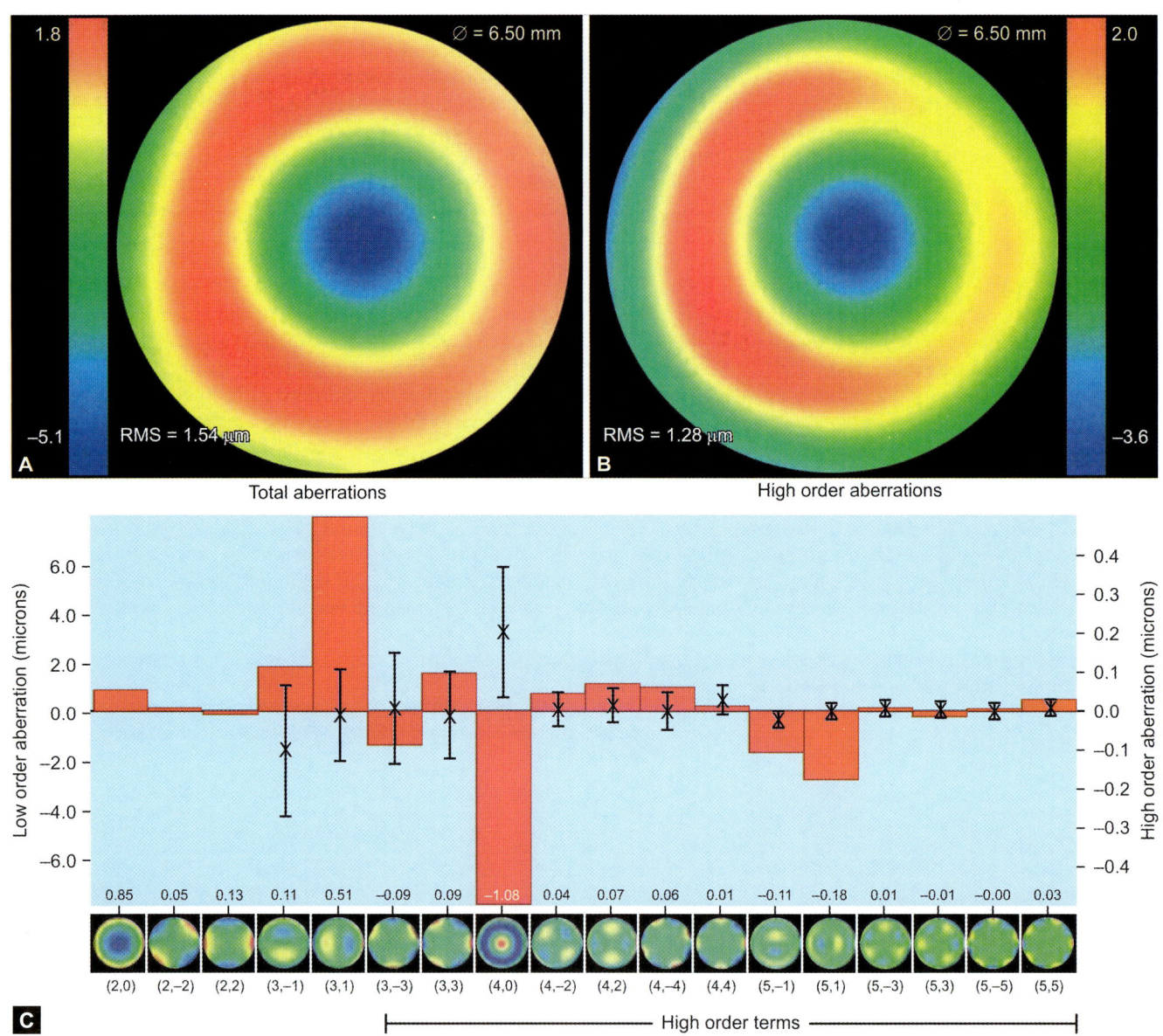

Figs 2A to C: Preoperative wavefront maps of (A) right and (B) left eyes reveal dominant spherical aberrations in both eyes, represented by a highly negative center with positive ring; (C) Zernike modes, including coma and spherical, with patient's total-eye aberration values are shown below wavefront maps

abnormalities that first went undetected by other ophthalmic examinations, including anterior segment slit-lamp. Eye aberrations can result from both lenticular and corneal imperfections since the cornea and lens contribute approximately two-thirds and one-third of the total focusing power of the eye, respectively. The subtlety of the lenticular abnormality made it difficult to detect and was only observed after wavefront analysis first pointed to it as a contributing factor in the patient's vision loss.

Wavefront maps define the deviation of an aberrated wavefront from the ideal reference wavefront. The reference shape used for comparison is a flat, circular plane which represents an emmetropic, or theoretically perfect, eye. RMS values correspond to decreases in optical quality and are represented by deviations from the emmetropic plane as cooler or warmer colors. Evaluation of higher-order aberrations in our patient revealed predominant spherical aberration in both eyes **(Figs 2A to C)**, suggesting

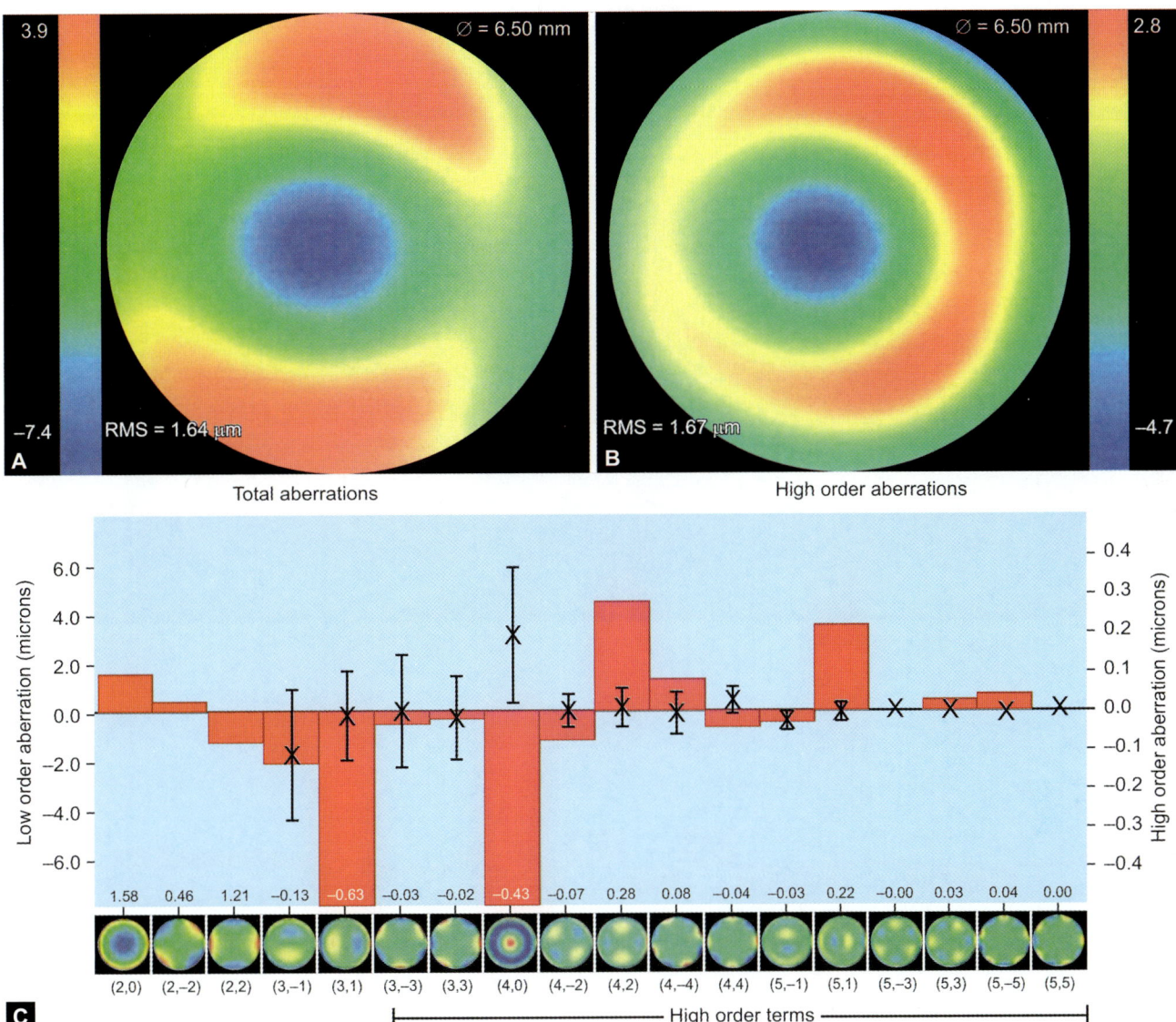

Figs 3A to C: Scheimpflug images distinguishing the dilated lens contour of anterior lenticonus (A) and that of a normal lens (B). (C) 4 mm chord and lens protrusion values are indicated

that reflection patterns were produced by an anterior lens surface bulge. In a study evaluating irregular astigmatism, Ninomoya and associates[6] found that astigmatism induced by anterior lenticonus produced such spherical-like aberrations. On the other hand, predominance of coma-like aberrations would have indicated keratoconus-induced irregular astigmatism.

Further examination with the Scheimpflug camera captured a complete picture of the anterior segment and provided visual confirmation of AL. Measurements and calculations performed on the images supported the diagnosis with quantitative results. Lenticular protrusion at 400 μm from a 4 mm chord was more than three standard deviations away from the mean of fifteen normal patients at 256.7 μm. Given the patient's medical history of Alport syndrome and wavefront analysis results, Scheimpflug imaging was sufficient to confirm the diagnosis.

After cataract extraction and IOL implantation, total-eye aberrations were reduced from 2.64 μm to 1.38 μm. The improvements in optical quality are reflected in the postoperative wavefront map and aberration values (**Figs 4A to C**), which show a much greater resemblance to a flat,

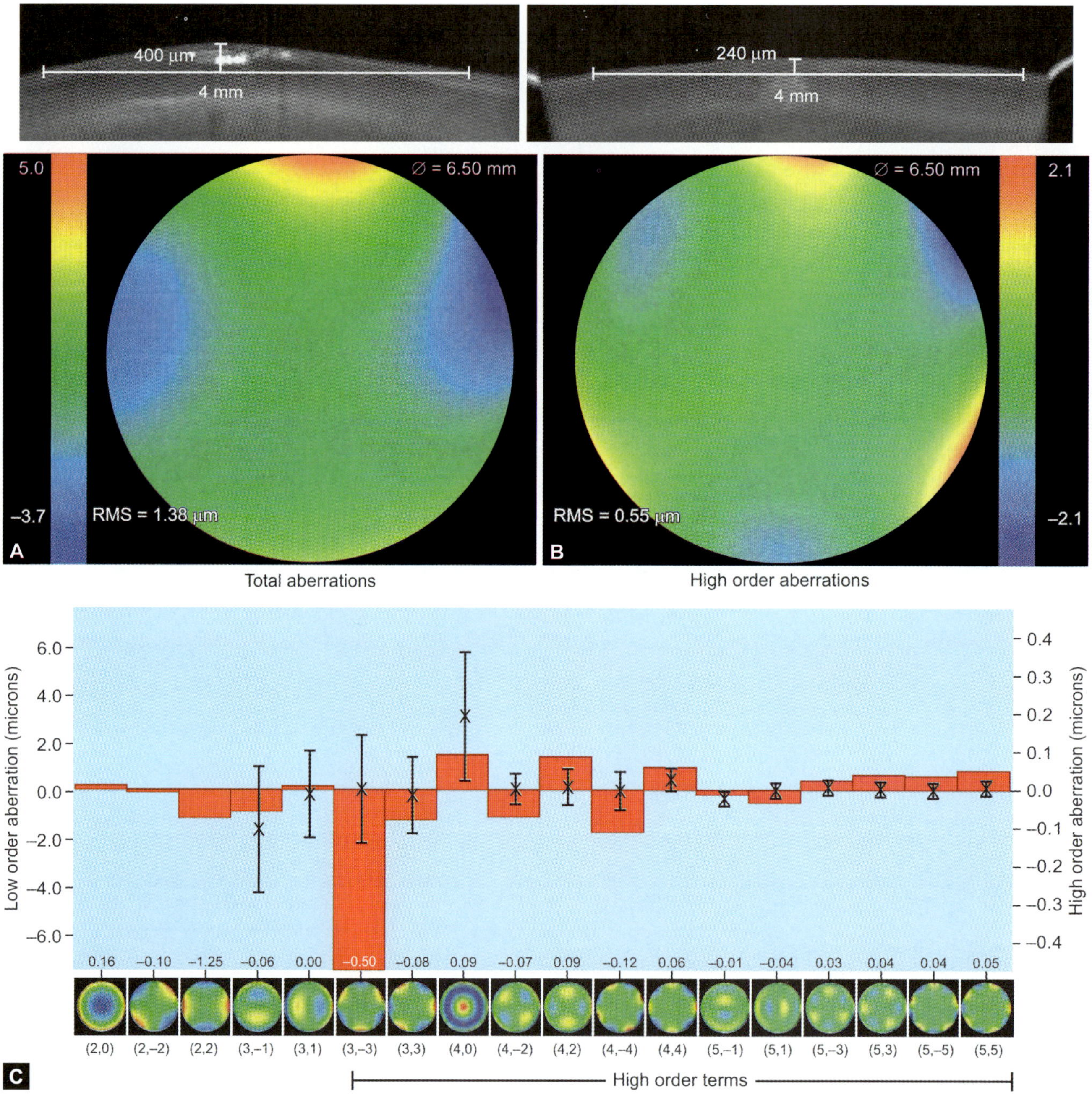

Figs 4A to C: Postoperative wavefront maps (A and B) and Zernike modes (C) of left eye showing significant reduction of spherical and other aberrations, resulting in a greater resemblance to the emmetropic eye

circular plane, representing the emmetropic eye. As most of the aberrations were due to lenticonus, surgical treatment dramatically restored the patient's left eye vision from $20/40^{-2}$ to a BCVA of 20/25.

Advanced imaging technologies are useful for diagnosing a variety of optical disorders, including anterior lenticonus.

Since optical disorders may be of various origins, such as lenticular, corneal, retinal and/or neurological, a long differential process of elimination may be required. However, wavefront analysis can assist the diagnostic process by identifying subtle abnormalities through characteristic clues such as spherical and coma aberrations. Finally, when correlated with medical history and wavefront analysis, Scheimpflug imaging can provide visual confirmation of treatable pathology.

REFERENCES

1. Blaise P, Delanaye P, Martalo O, Pierard GE, Rorive G, Galand A. Anterior lenticonus: diagnostic aid in Alport syndrome. J Fr Ophtalmol. 2003;26:1075-82.
2. Liu YB, Tan SJ, Sun ZY, Li X, Huang BY, Hu QM. Clear lens phacoemulsification with continuous curvilinear capsulorhexis and foldable intraocular lens implantation for the treatment of a patient with bilateral anterior lenticonus due to Alport syndrome. J Int Med Res. 2008;36:1440-4.
3. Lagona E, Tsartsali L, Kostaridou S, Skiathitou A, Georgaki E, Sotsiou F. Skin biopsy for the diagnosis of Alport Syndrome. Hippokratia. 2008;12:116-8.
4. Amiraslanzadeh G. Is anterior lenticonus the most common ocular finding in Alport syndrome? J Cataract Refract Surg. 2008;34:5.
5. Grewal DS, Jain R, Brar GS, Grewal SP. Scheimpflug imaging of pediatric posterior capsule rupture. Indian J Ophthalmol. 2009;57:236-8.
6. Ninomoya S, Maeda N, Kuroda T. Evaluation of lenticular irregular astigmatism using wavefront analysis in patients with lenticonus. Arch Ophthalmol. 2002;120:1388-93.

CHAPTER 10

CHAPTER 11

Roberto Pinelli

P-curve Clinical Cases

P-curve^{TM} is an algorithm patented for correcting presbyopia through LASIK.

The cases show aberrations changes after P-curve ablations. All the cases show presbyopia correction with J1 OU in all the patients.

A short analysis of aberrations changes shows negative spherical aberrations augmentation in ALL cases.

This probably means that negative spherical aberrations have a rule in presbyopia correction.

Do not forget that, in any human being eye, accommodating, the negative spherical aberrations are growing in terms of number.

This means a simple thing negative spherical aberration is a key for presbyopia correction in a presbyopic patient.

Enjoy those clinical cases and think about the negative spherical aberration rule!

CASE 1: Female, 51 years old

Preoperative UCVA for Far

RE: 20/50 nat
LE: 20/50 nat

Preoperative UCVA for Near

RE: J6 nat
LE: J6 nat

Preoperative BCVA for Far

RE: 20/20 sph. +1.00
LE: 20/20 sph. + 0.75 cyl + 0.50 ax 85°

Preoperative BCVA for Near

J1 add. + 1.50 OU

Postoperative UCVA for Far (12 Months)

RE: 20/20
LE: 20/20

Autorefractometry Postoperative

RE: sph 0.00 cyl −0.50 ax 150°
LE: sph 0.00 cyl −0.75 ax 22°

Postoperative UCVA for Near

J1 OU.

CHAPTER 11

RE = Right Eye; LE = Left Eye; UCVA = Uncorrected Visual Acuity;
BCVA = Best-corrected Visual Acuity

Right Eye Preoperative Aberrations Map

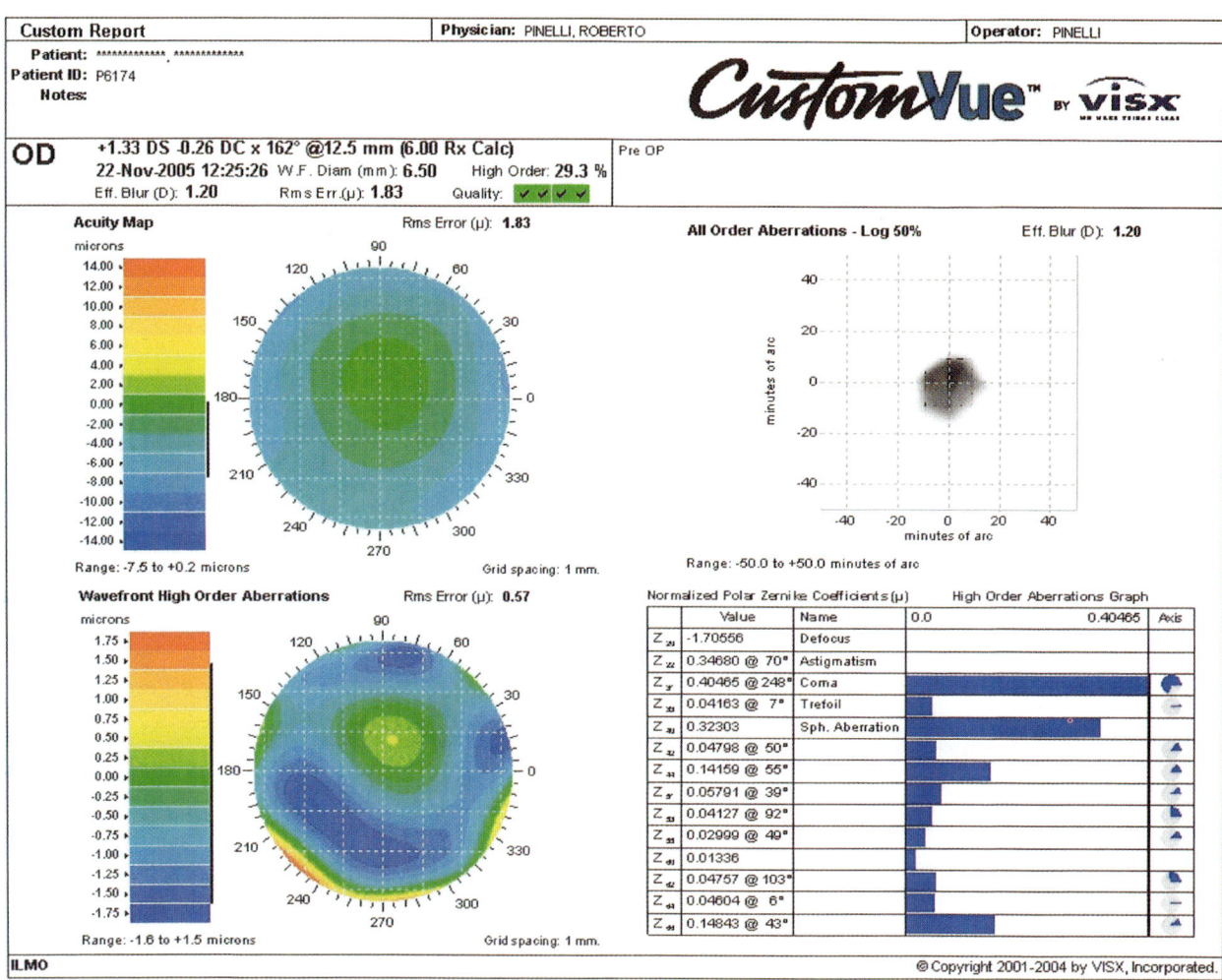

Right Eye Postoperative Aberrations Map

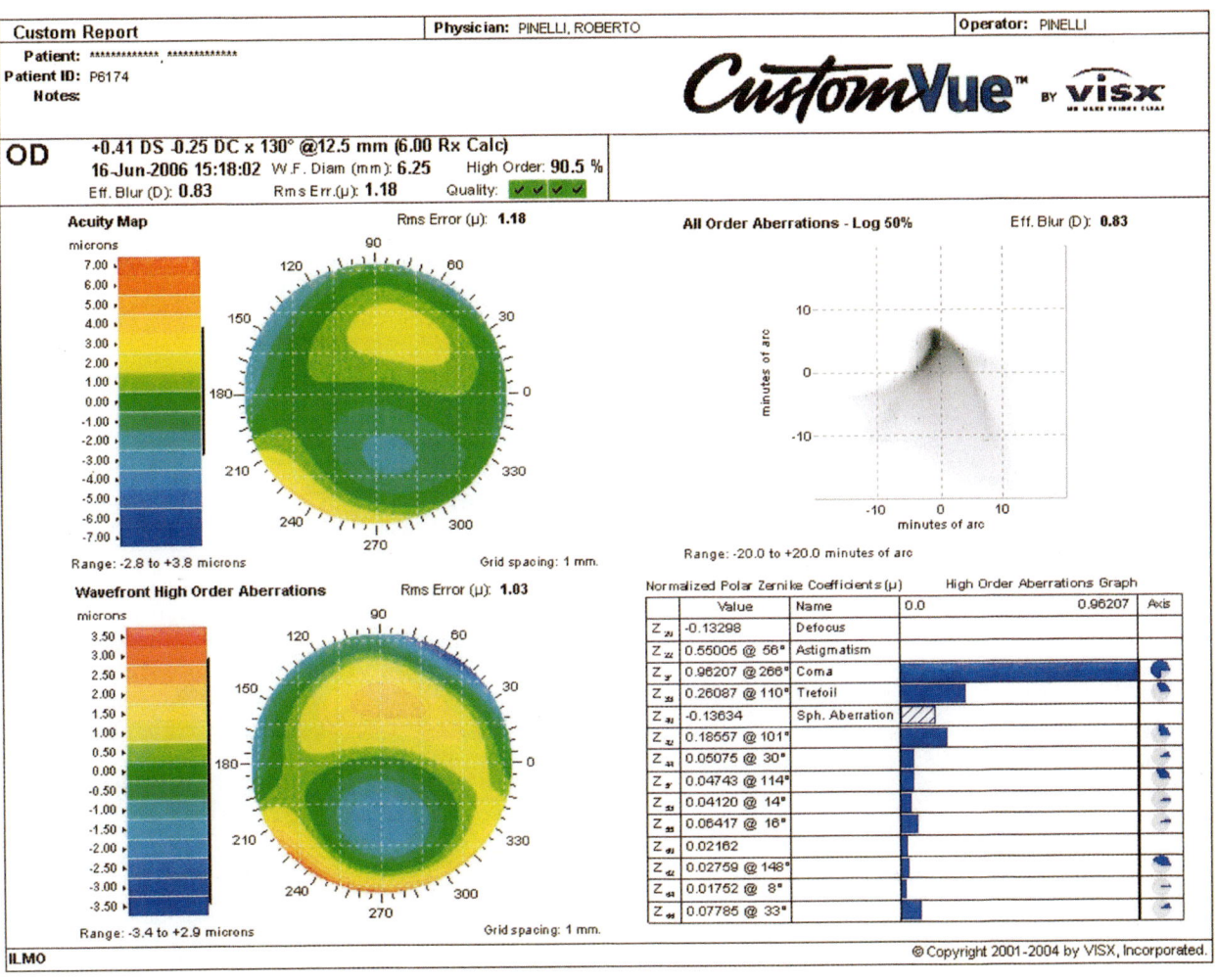

Custom Report		Physician: PINELLI, ROBERTO	Operator: PINELLI

Patient: **************, ************
Patient ID: P6174
Notes:

OD +0.41 DS -0.25 DC x 130° @12.5 mm (6.00 Rx Calc)
16-Jun-2006 15:18:02 W.F. Diam (mm): 6.25   High Order: 90.5 %
Eff. Blur (D): 0.83   Rms Err.(µ): 1.18   Quality: ✓✓✓

Acuity Map   Rms Error (µ): 1.18

microns
7.00
6.00
5.00
4.00
3.00
2.00
1.00
0.00
-1.00
-2.00
-3.00
-4.00
-5.00
-6.00
-7.00

Range: -2.8 to +3.8 microns   Grid spacing: 1 mm.

All Order Aberrations - Log 50%   Eff. Blur (D): 0.83

Range: -20.0 to +20.0 minutes of arc

Wavefront High Order Aberrations   Rms Error (µ): 1.03

microns
3.50
3.00
2.50
2.00
1.50
1.00
0.50
0.00
-0.50
-1.00
-1.50
-2.00
-2.50
-3.00
-3.50

Range: -3.4 to +2.9 microns   Grid spacing: 1 mm.

Normalized Polar Zernike Coefficients (µ)   High Order Aberrations Graph

	Value	Name	0.0	0.96207	Axis
Z_{20}	-0.13298	Defocus			
Z_{22}	0.55005 @ 56°	Astigmatism			
Z_{3f}	0.96207 @ 266°	Coma			
Z_{33}	0.26087 @ 110°	Trefoil			
Z_{40}	-0.13634	Sph. Aberration			
Z_{42}	0.18557 @ 101°				
Z_{44}	0.05075 @ 30°				
Z_{5f}	0.04743 @ 114°				
Z_{53}	0.04120 @ 14°				
Z_{55}	0.06417 @ 16°				
Z_{60}	0.02162				
Z_{62}	0.02759 @ 148°				
Z_{64}	0.01752 @ 8°				
Z_{66}	0.07785 @ 33°				

ILMO

Left Eye Preoperative Aberrations Map

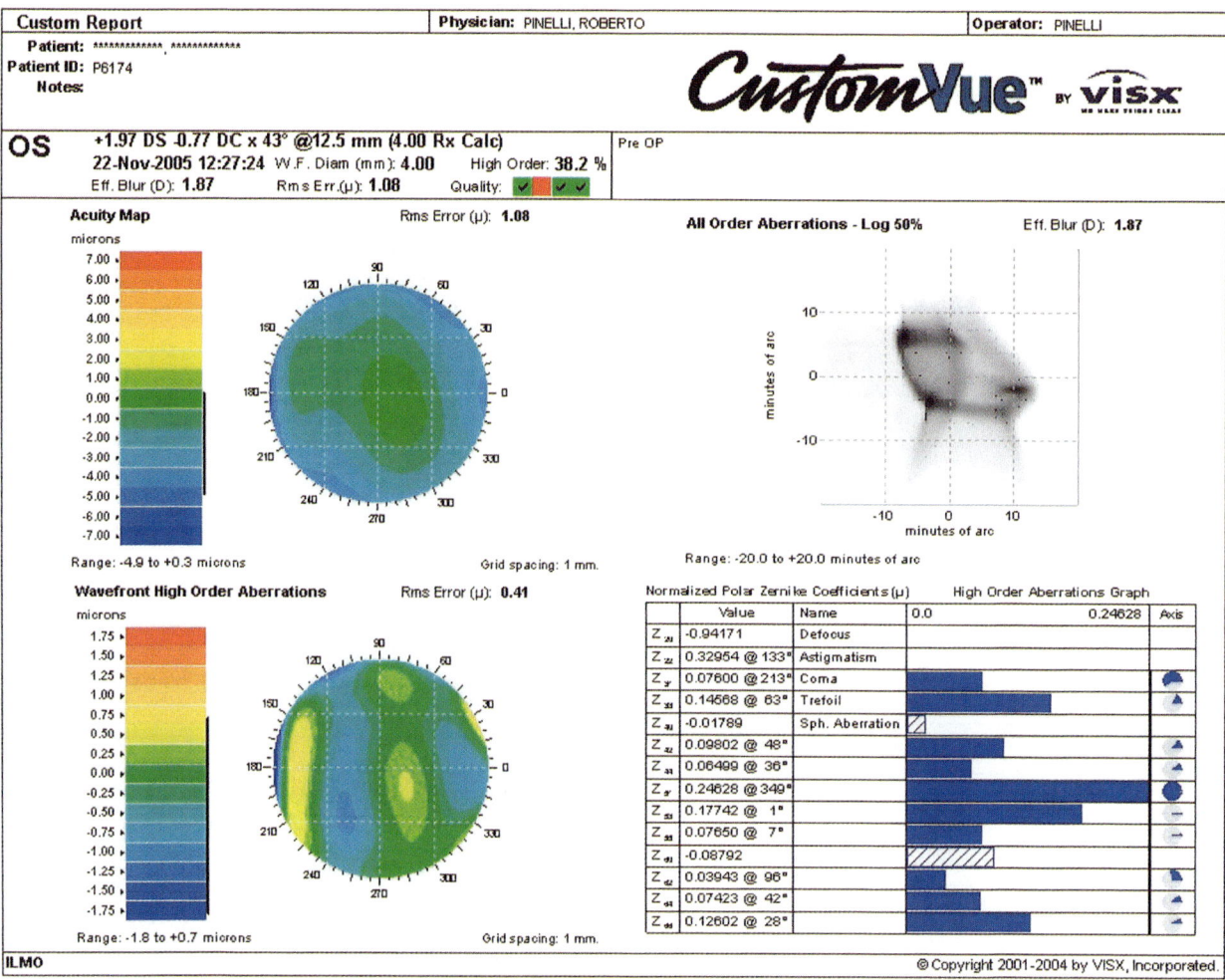

3
SECTION

Left Eye Postoperative Aberrations Map

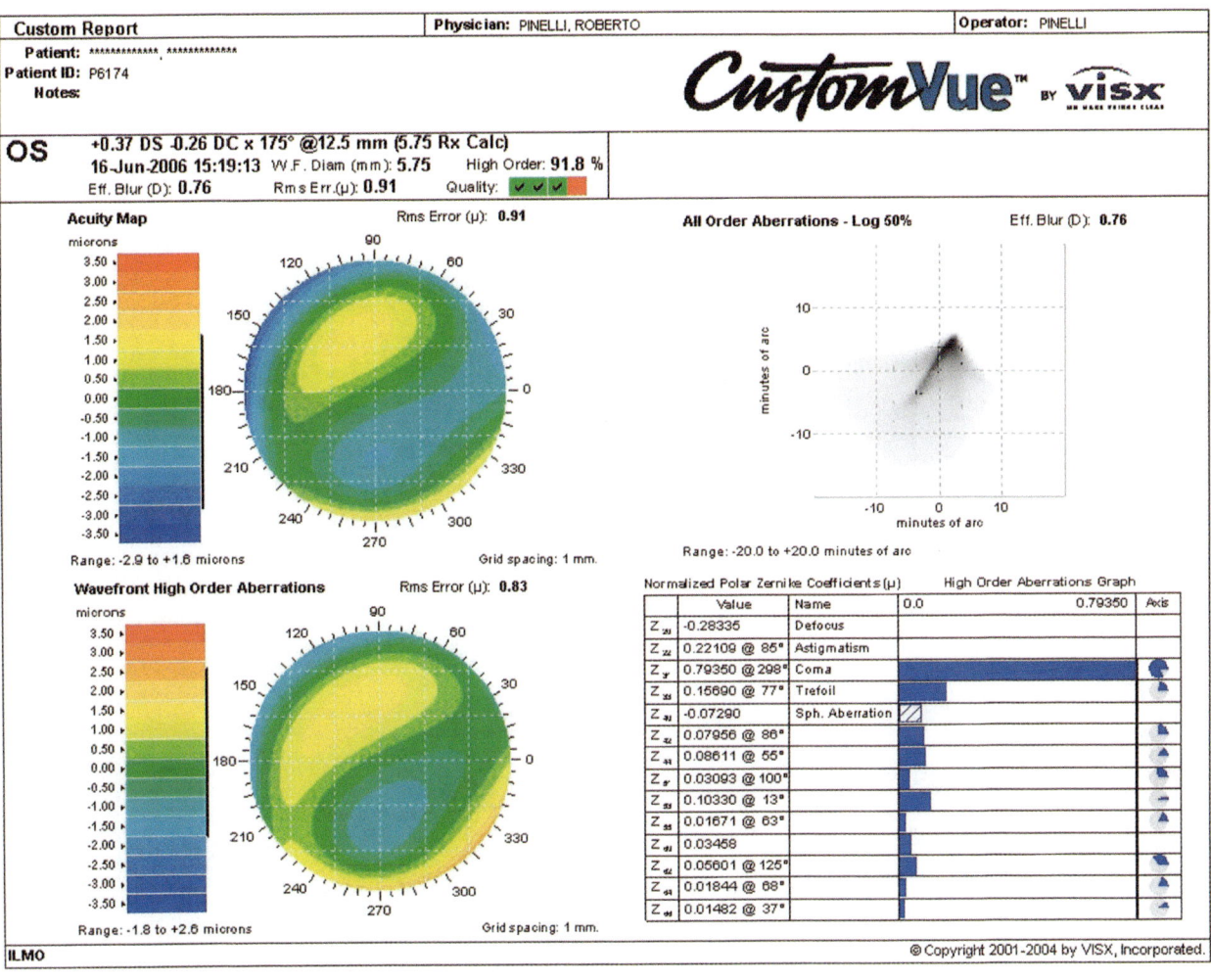

	Value	Name	0.0	0.79350	Axis
Z_{20}	-0.28335	Defocus			
Z_{22}	0.22109 @ 85°	Astigmatism			
Z_{3f}	0.79350 @ 298°	Coma			
Z_{33}	0.15690 @ 77°	Trefoil			
Z_{40}	-0.07290	Sph. Aberration			
Z_{42}	0.07956 @ 86°				
Z_{44}	0.08611 @ 55°				
Z_{5f}	0.03093 @ 100°				
Z_{53}	0.10330 @ 13°				
Z_{55}	0.01671 @ 63°				
Z_{60}	0.03458				
Z_{62}	0.05601 @ 125°				
Z_{64}	0.01844 @ 68°				
Z_{66}	0.01482 @ 37°				

CASE 2: Female, 55 years old

Preoperative UCVA for Far

RE: 20/40 nat
LE: 20/40 nat

Preoperative UCVA for Near

RE: J7 nat
LE: J7 nat

Preoperative BCVA for Far

RE: 20/20 sph. +0.50 Cyl 0.50 ax 90°
LE: 20/20 sph. +0.50 cyl +1.00 ax 80°

Preoperative BCVA for Near

J1 add. +1.75 OU

Postoperative UCVA for Far (12 Months)

RE: 20/20
LE: 20/20

Autorefractometry Postoperative

RE: sph 0.00 cyl −0.25 ax 65°
LE: sph +0.50 cyl +0.50 ax 15°

Postoperative UCVA for Near

J1 OU.

Right Eye Preoperative Aberrations Map

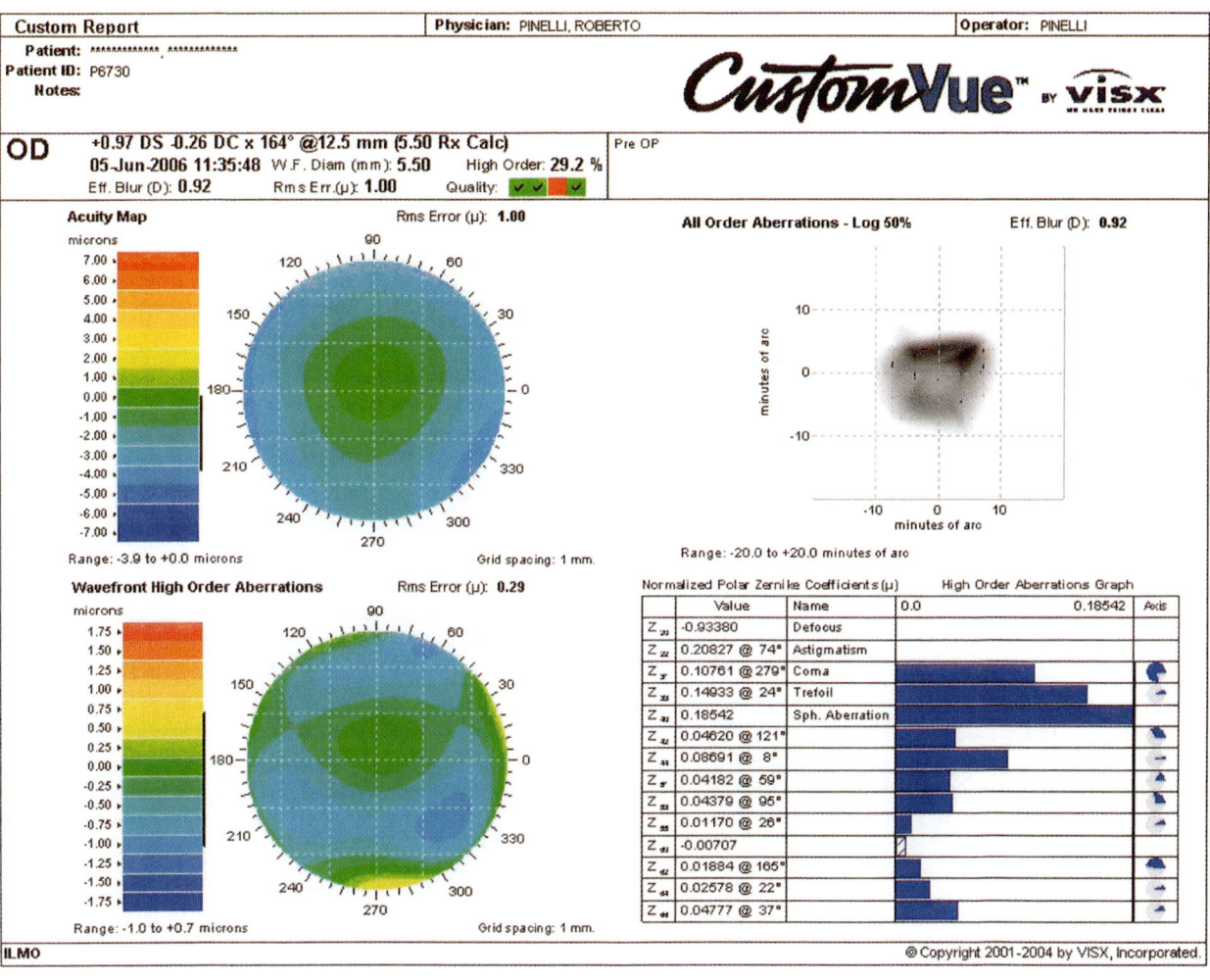

Right Eye Postoperative Aberrations Map

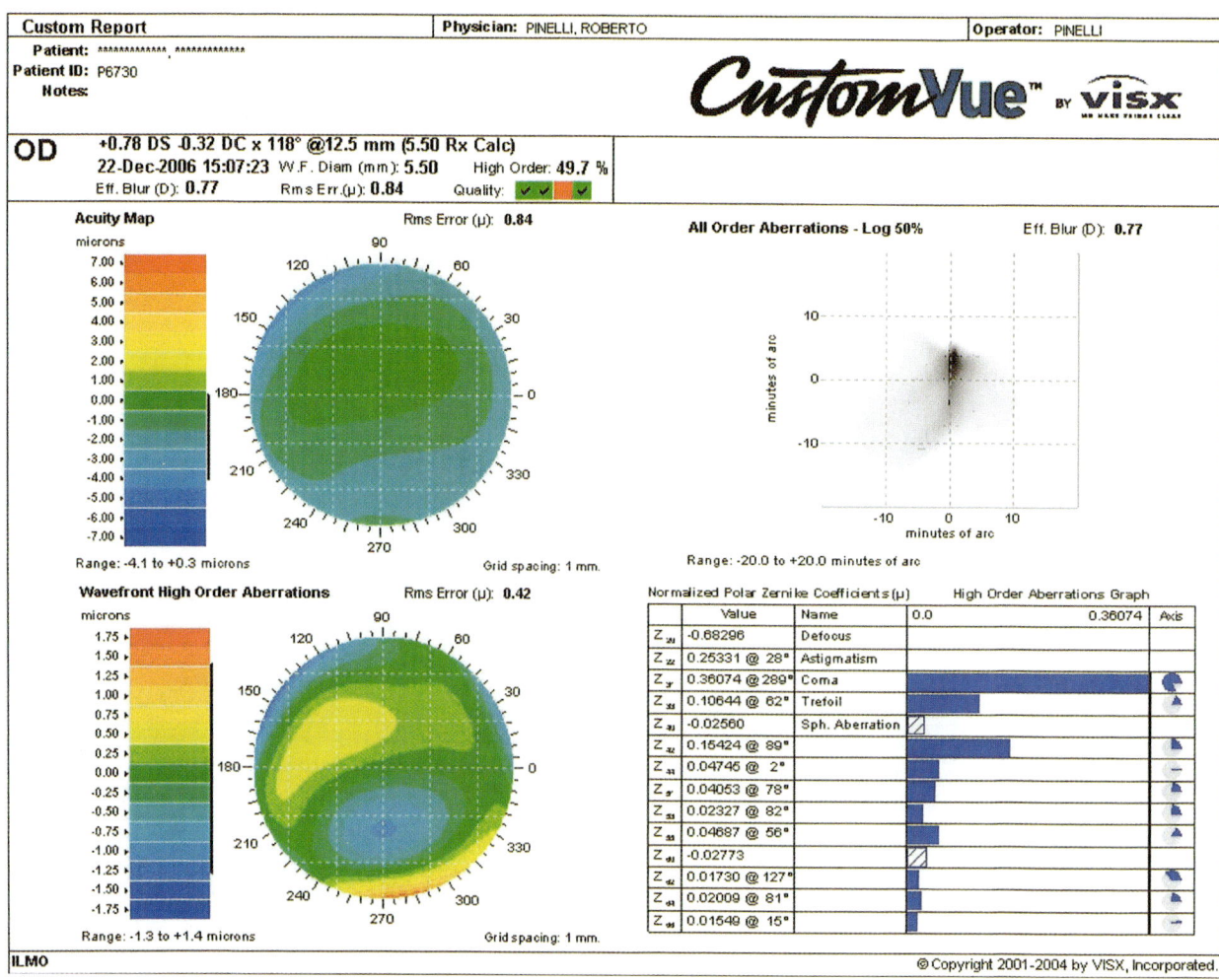

Custom Report	Physician: PINELLI, ROBERTO	Operator: PINELLI

Patient: ^^^^^^^^^^^^^^^, ^^^^^^^^^^^^^^^
Patient ID: P6730
Notes:

CustomVue™ BY **visx** WE MAKE THINGS CLEAR

OD   +0.78 DS -0.32 DC x 118° @12.5 mm (5.50 Rx Calc)
22-Dec-2006 15:07:23   W.F. Diam (mm): **5.50**   High Order: **49.7 %**
Eff. Blur (D): **0.77**   Rms Err.(µ): **0.84**   Quality: ✔✔▇✔

Acuity Map   Rms Error (µ): 0.84

microns
7.00
6.00
5.00
4.00
3.00
2.00
1.00
0.00
-1.00
-2.00
-3.00
-4.00
-5.00
-6.00
-7.00

Range: -4.1 to +0.3 microns   Grid spacing: 1 mm.

All Order Aberrations - Log 50%   Eff. Blur (D): 0.77

minutes of arc

Range: -20.0 to +20.0 minutes of arc

Wavefront High Order Aberrations   Rms Error (µ): 0.42

microns
1.75
1.50
1.25
1.00
0.75
0.50
0.25
0.00
-0.25
-0.50
-0.75
-1.00
-1.25
-1.50
-1.75

Range: -1.3 to +1.4 microns   Grid spacing: 1 mm.

Normalized Polar Zernike Coefficients (µ)   High Order Aberrations Graph

	Value	Name	0.0	0.36074	Axis
Z_{20}	-0.68296	Defocus			
Z_{22}	0.25331 @ 28°	Astigmatism			
Z_{31}	0.36074 @ 289°	Coma			
Z_{33}	0.10644 @ 62°	Trefoil			
Z_{40}	-0.02560	Sph. Aberration			
Z_{42}	0.15424 @ 89°				
Z_{44}	0.04745 @ 2°				
Z_{51}	0.04053 @ 78°				
Z_{53}	0.02327 @ 82°				
Z_{55}	0.04687 @ 56°				
Z_{60}	-0.02773				
Z_{62}	0.01730 @ 127°				
Z_{64}	0.02009 @ 81°				
Z_{66}	0.01549 @ 15°				

ILMO   © Copyright 2001-2004 by VISX, Incorporated.

Left Eye Preoperative Aberrations Map

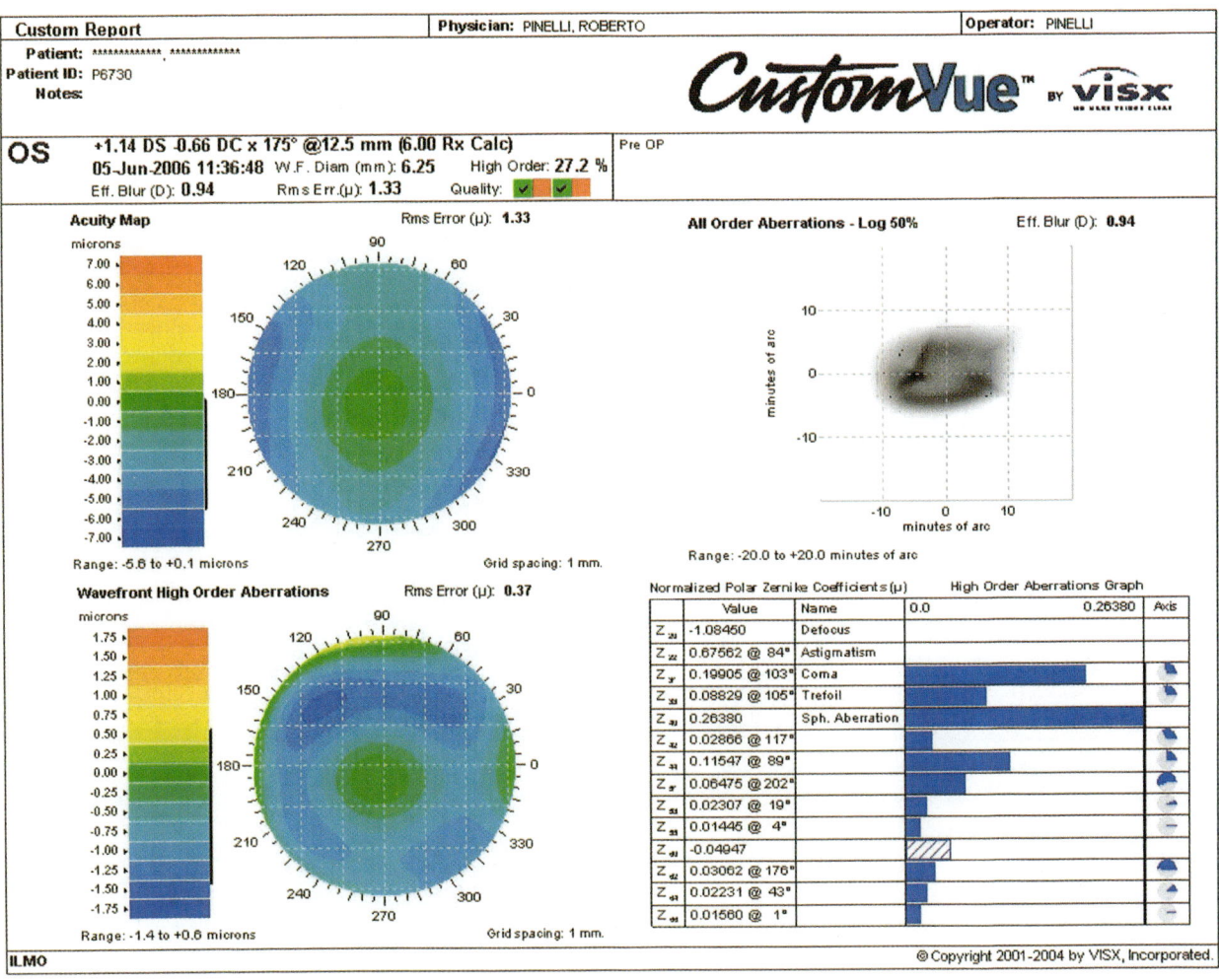

	Value	Name	0.0	0.26380	Axis
Z_{20}	-1.08450	Defocus			
Z_{22}	0.67562 @ 84°	Astigmatism			
Z_{3f}	0.19905 @ 103°	Coma			
Z_{33}	0.08829 @ 105°	Trefoil			
Z_{4f}	0.26380	Sph. Aberration			
Z_{42}	0.02866 @ 117°				
Z_{4f}	0.11547 @ 89°				
Z_{4f}	0.06475 @ 202°				
Z_{4f}	0.02307 @ 19°				
Z_{5f}	0.01445 @ 4°				
Z_{4f}	-0.04947				
Z_{4f}	0.03062 @ 176°				
Z_{4f}	0.02231 @ 43°				
Z_{4f}	0.01560 @ 1°				

ILMO

© Copyright 2001-2004 by VISX, Incorporated.

3 SECTION

Left Eye Postoperative Aberrations Map

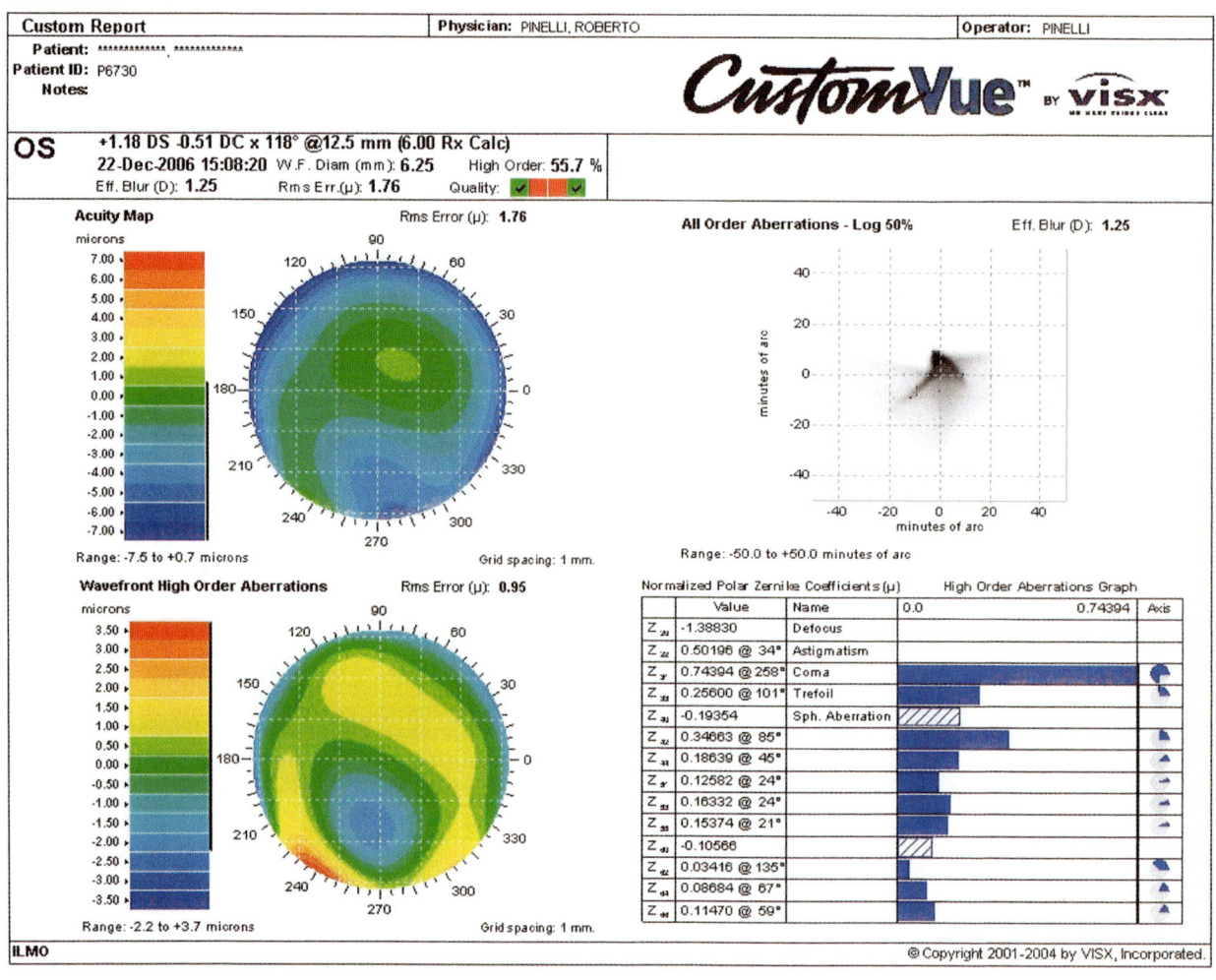

Custom Report	Physician: PINELLI, ROBERTO	Operator: PINELLI

Patient: ************ ************
Patient ID: P6730
Notes:

CustomVue™ BY **visx**

OS +1.18 DS -0.51 DC x 118° @12.5 mm (6.00 Rx Calc)
22-Dec-2006 15:08:20 W.F. Diam (mm): **6.25**   High Order: **55.7 %**
Eff. Blur (D): **1.25**   Rms Err.(µ): **1.76**   Quality:

Acuity Map   Rms Error (µ): **1.76**
microns
7.00 · 6.00 · 5.00 · 4.00 · 3.00 · 2.00 · 1.00 · 0.00 · -1.00 · -2.00 · -3.00 · -4.00 · -5.00 · -6.00 · -7.00
Range: -7.5 to +0.7 microns   Grid spacing: 1 mm.

Wavefront High Order Aberrations   Rms Error (µ): **0.95**
microns
3.50 · 3.00 · 2.50 · 2.00 · 1.50 · 1.00 · 0.50 · 0.00 · -0.50 · -1.00 · -1.50 · -2.00 · -2.50 · -3.00 · -3.50
Range: -2.2 to +3.7 microns   Grid spacing: 1 mm.

All Order Aberrations - Log 50%   Eff. Blur (D): **1.25**
Range: -50.0 to +50.0 minutes of arc

Normalized Polar Zernike Coefficients (µ)   High Order Aberrations Graph

	Value	Name	0.0	0.74394	Axis
Z_{20}	-1.38830	Defocus			
Z_{22}	0.50196 @ 34°	Astigmatism			
Z_{31}	0.74394 @ 258°	Coma			
Z_{33}	0.25600 @ 101°	Trefoil			
Z_{40}	-0.19354	Sph. Aberration			
Z_{42}	0.34663 @ 85°				
Z_{44}	0.18639 @ 45°				
Z_{51}	0.12582 @ 24°				
Z_{53}	0.16332 @ 24°				
Z_{55}	0.15374 @ 21°				
Z_{60}	-0.10566				
Z_{62}	0.03416 @ 135°				
Z_{64}	0.08684 @ 67°				
Z_{66}	0.11470 @ 59°				

ILMO   © Copyright 2001-2004 by VISX, Incorporated.

CASE 3: Female, 50 years old

Preoperative UCVA for Far

RE: 20/32 nat
LE: 20/32 nat

Preoperative UCVA for Near

RE: J6 nat
LE: J6 nat

Preoperative BCVA for Far

RE: 20/20 sph. + 0.00 cyl + 1.00 ax 90°
LE: 20/20 sph. + 0.00 cyl + 0.50 ax 90°

Preoperative BCVA for Near

J1 add. +1.25 OU

Postoperative UCVA for Far (12 Months)

RE: 20/20
LE: 20/20

Autorefractometry Postoperative

RE: sph + 0.50 cyl –0.75 ax 30°
LE: sph –0.25 cyl –0.50 ax 160°

Postoperative UCVA for Near

J1 OU.

Right Eye Preoperative Aberrations Map

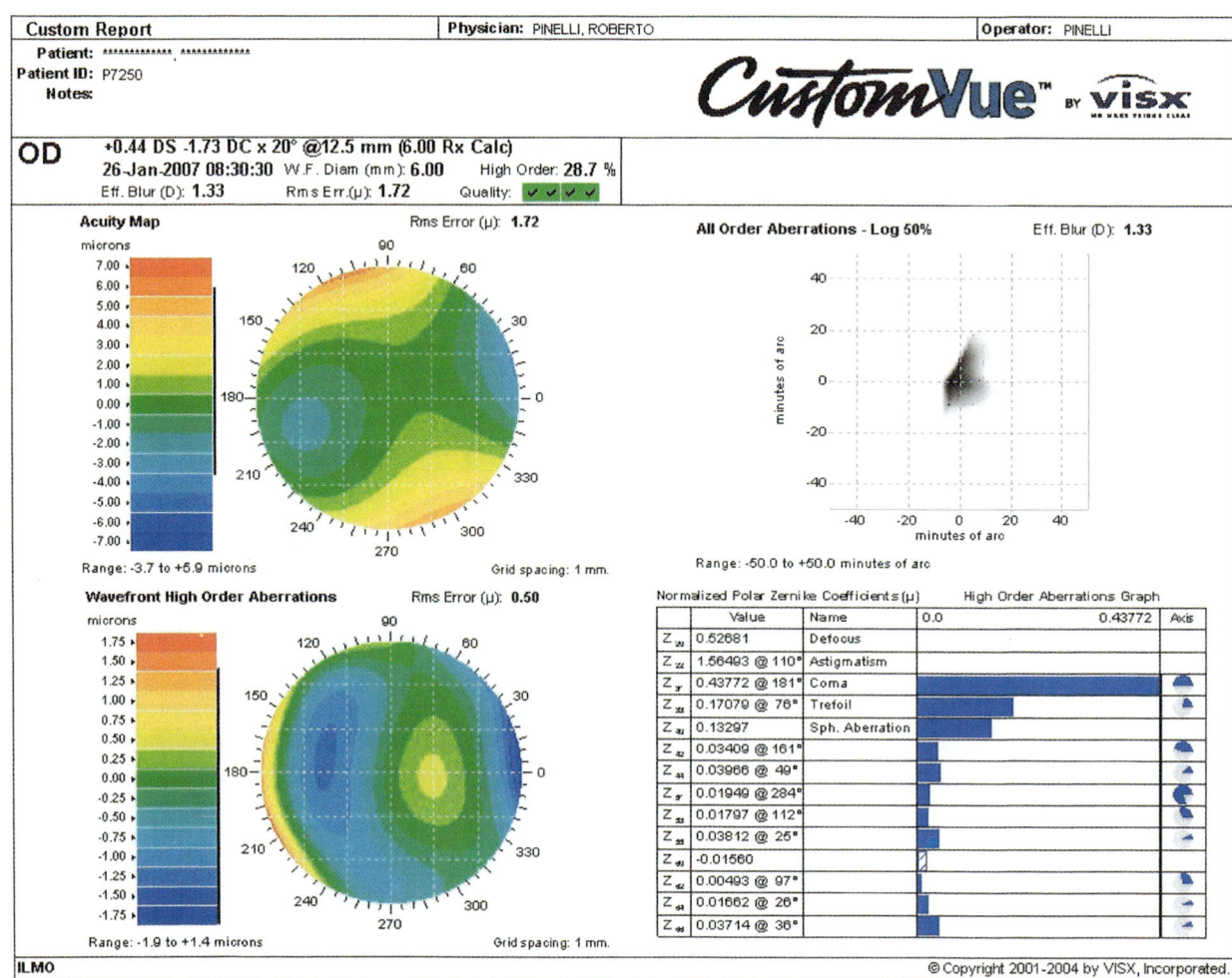

	Value	Name	0.0	0.43772	Axis
Z_{20}	0.52681	Defocus			
Z_{22}	1.56493 @ 110°	Astigmatism			
Z_{3f}	0.43772 @ 181°	Coma			
Z_{33}	0.17079 @ 76°	Trefoil			
Z_{40}	0.13297	Sph. Aberration			
Z_{42}	0.03409 @ 161°				
Z_{3f}	0.03966 @ 49°				
Z_{3f}	0.01949 @ 284°				
Z_{43}	0.01797 @ 112°				
Z_{53}	0.03812 @ 25°				
Z_{6f}	-0.01560				
Z_{6f}	0.00493 @ 97°				
Z_{66}	0.01662 @ 26°				
Z_{66}	0.03714 @ 36°				

ILMO

Right Eye Postoperative Aberrations Map

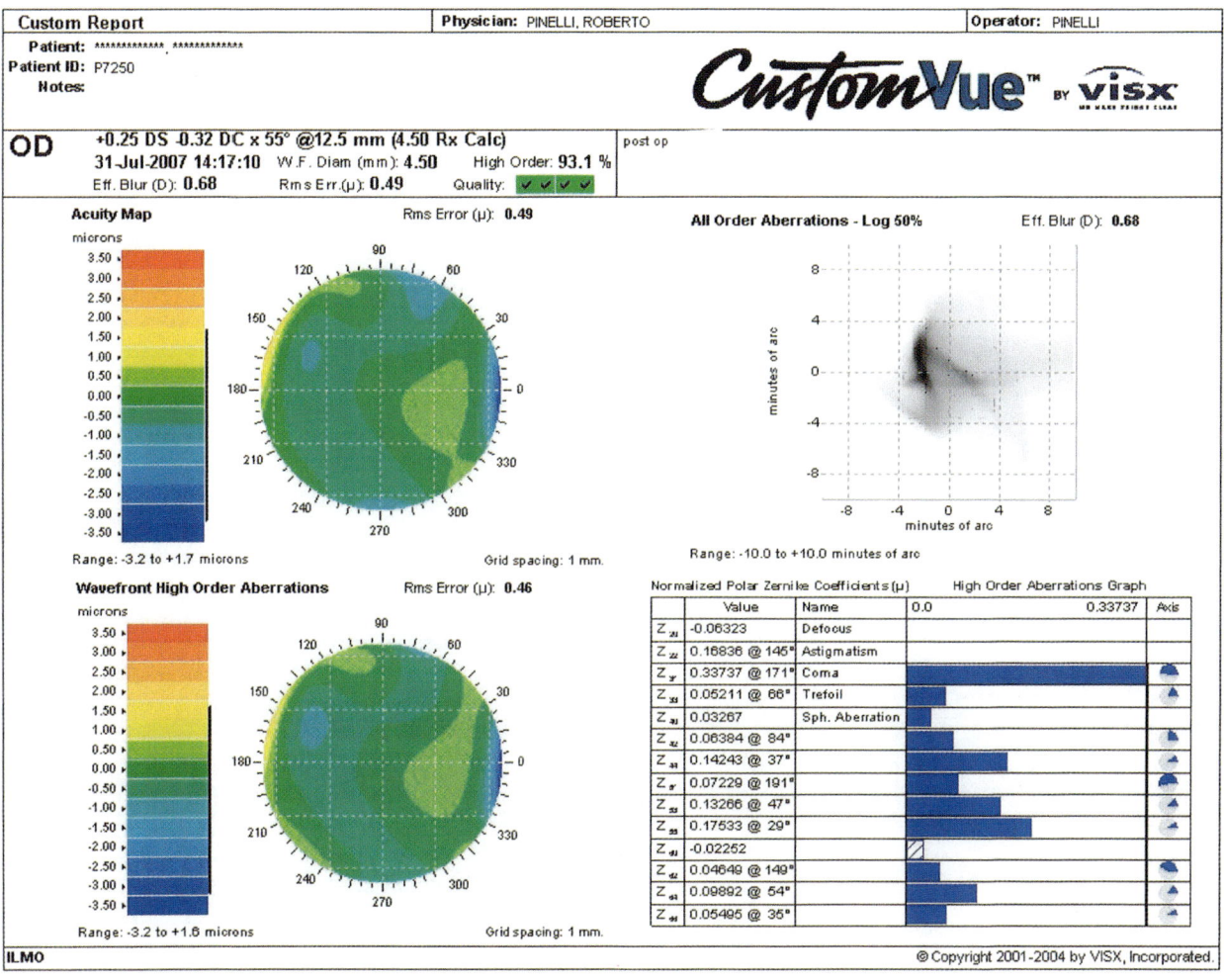

Normalized Polar Zernike Coefficients (µ) — High Order Aberrations Graph

	Value	Name	0.0	0.33737	Axis
Z_{20}	-0.06323	Defocus			
Z_{22}	0.16836 @ 145°	Astigmatism			
Z_{31}	0.33737 @ 171°	Coma			
Z_{33}	0.05211 @ 66°	Trefoil			
Z_{40}	0.03267	Sph. Aberration			
Z_{42}	0.06384 @ 84°				
Z_{44}	0.14243 @ 37°				
Z_{51}	0.07229 @ 191°				
Z_{53}	0.13266 @ 47°				
Z_{55}	0.17533 @ 29°				
Z_{60}	-0.02252				
Z_{62}	0.04649 @ 149°				
Z_{64}	0.09892 @ 54°				
Z_{66}	0.05495 @ 35°				

ILMO

Left Eye Preoperative Aberrations Map

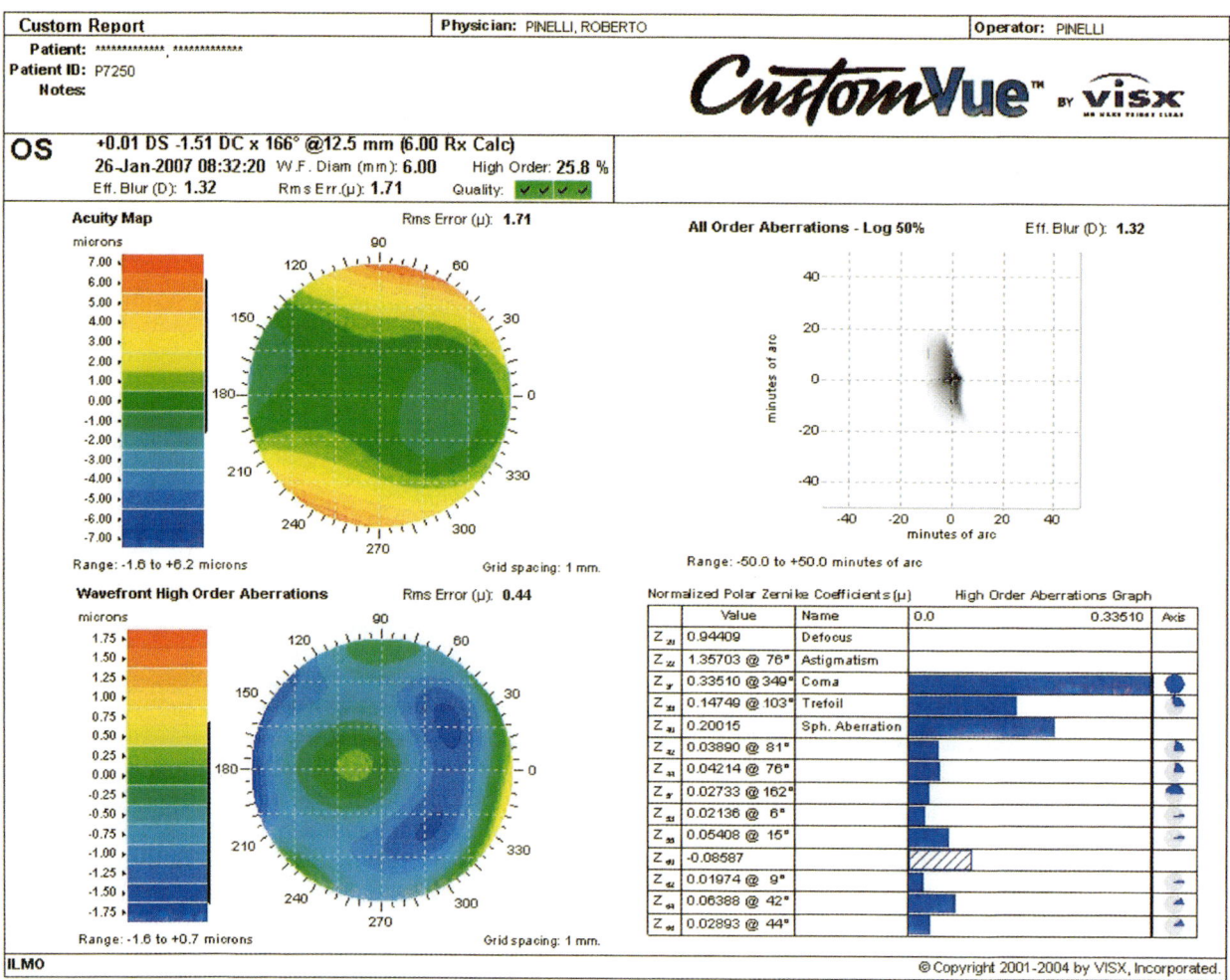

SECTION 3

	Value	Name	0.0	0.33510	Axis
Z_{20}	0.94409	Defocus			
Z_{22}	1.35703 @ 76°	Astigmatism			
Z_{31}	0.33510 @ 349°	Coma			
Z_{33}	0.14749 @ 103°	Trefoil			
Z_{40}	0.20015	Sph. Aberration			
Z_{42}	0.03890 @ 81°				
Z_{44}	0.04214 @ 76°				
Z_{51}	0.02733 @ 162°				
Z_{53}	0.02136 @ 6°				
Z_{55}	0.05408 @ 15°				
Z_{60}	-0.08587				
Z_{62}	0.01974 @ 9°				
Z_{64}	0.06388 @ 42°				
Z_{66}	0.02893 @ 44°				

ILMO

Left Eye Postoperative Aberrations Map

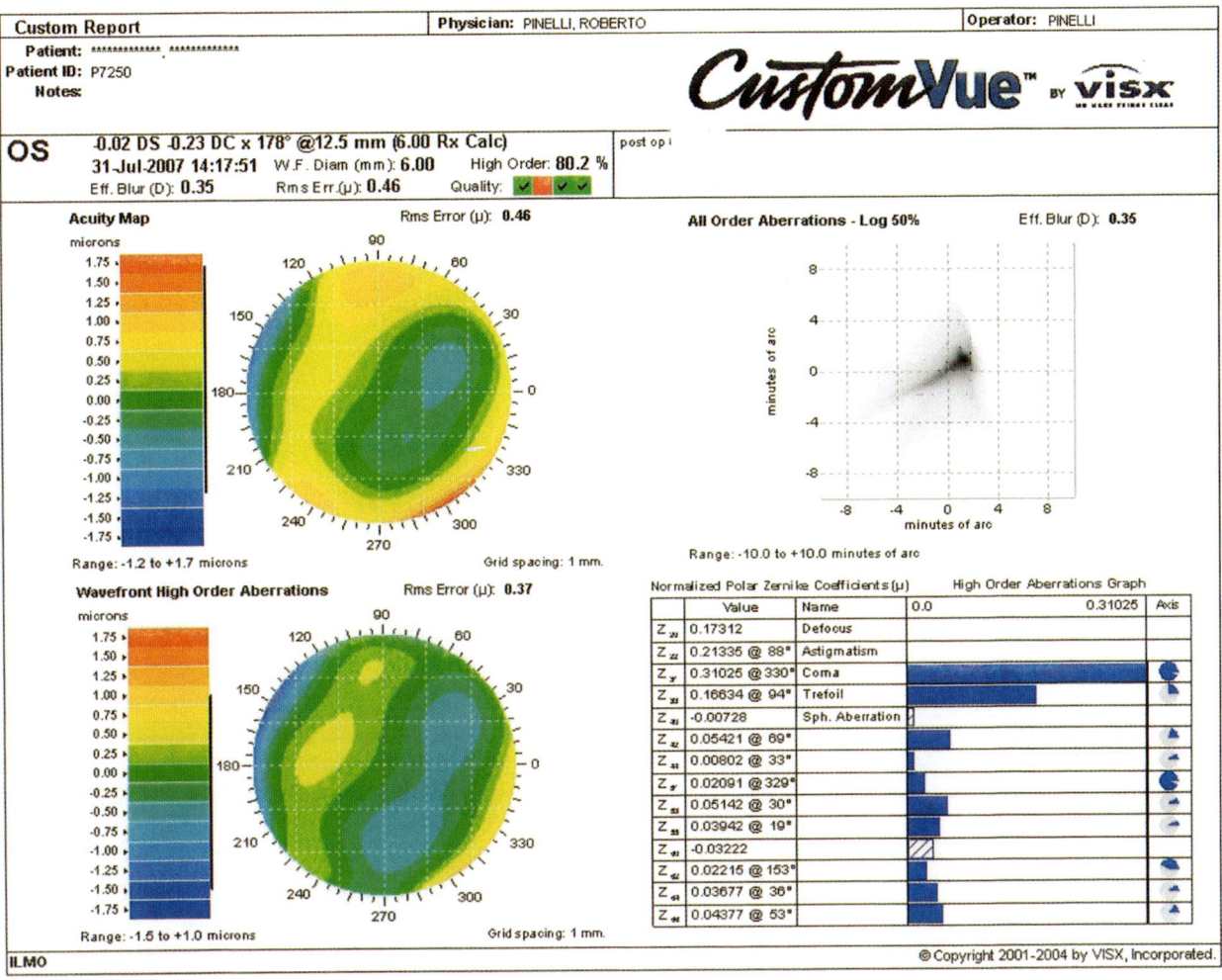

	Value	Name	0.0	0.31025	Axis
Z_{20}	0.17312	Defocus			
Z_{22}	0.21335 @ 88°	Astigmatism			
Z_{31}	0.31025 @ 330°	Coma			
Z_{33}	0.16634 @ 94°	Trefoil			
Z_{40}	-0.00728	Sph. Aberration			
Z_{42}	0.05421 @ 69°				
Z_{44}	0.00802 @ 33°				
Z_{51}	0.02091 @ 329°				
Z_{53}	0.05142 @ 30°				
Z_{55}	0.03942 @ 19°				
Z_{60}	-0.03222				
Z_{62}	0.02215 @ 153°				
Z_{64}	0.03677 @ 36°				
Z_{66}	0.04377 @ 53°				

CASE 4: Male, 53 years old

Preoperative UCVA for Far

RE: 20/40 nat
LE: 20/40 nat

Preoperative UCVA for Near

RE: J6 nat
LE: J6 nat

Preoperative BCVA for Far

RE: 20/20 sph. + 0.75 Cyl /
LE: 20/20 sph. +1.00 Cyl /

Preoperative BCVA for Near

J1 add. + 1.50 OU

Postoperative UCVA for Far (12 Months)

RE: 20/20
LE: 20/20

Autorefractometry Postoperative

RE: sph + 0.00 cyl −0.75 ax 40°
LE: sph + 0.25 cyl −0.75 ax 160°

Postoperative UCVA for Near

J1 OU.

Right Eye Preoperative Aberrations Map

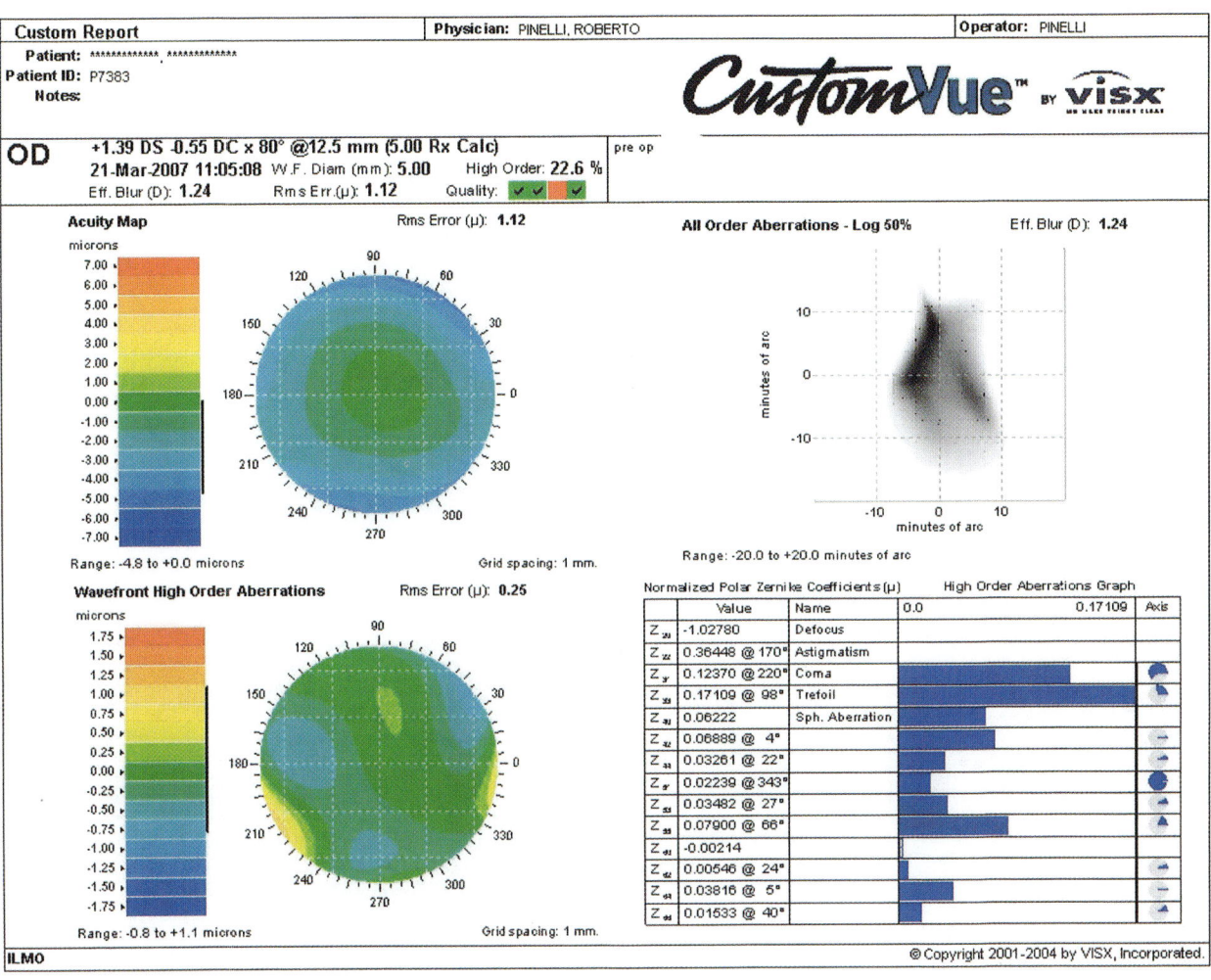

Custom Report		Physician: PINELLI, ROBERTO	Operator: PINELLI

Patient: ************* *************
Patient ID: P7383
Notes:

CustomVue™ BY **visx**

OD +1.39 DS -0.55 DC x 80° @12.5 mm (5.00 Rx Calc)   pre op
21-Mar-2007 11:05:08   W.F. Diam (mm): **5.00**   High Order: **22.6 %**
Eff. Blur (D): **1.24**   Rms Err.(µ): **1.12**   Quality: ✔ ✔ ▮ ✔

Acuity Map   Rms Error (µ): **1.12**

microns
7.00
6.00
5.00
4.00
3.00
2.00
1.00
0.00
-1.00
-2.00
-3.00
-4.00
-5.00
-6.00
-7.00

Range: -4.8 to +0.0 microns   Grid spacing: 1 mm.

All Order Aberrations - Log 50%   Eff. Blur (D): **1.24**

minutes of arc

Range: -20.0 to +20.0 minutes of arc

Wavefront High Order Aberrations   Rms Error (µ): **0.25**

microns
1.75
1.50
1.25
1.00
0.75
0.50
0.25
0.00
-0.25
-0.50
-0.75
-1.00
-1.25
-1.50
-1.75

Range: -0.8 to +1.1 microns   Grid spacing: 1 mm.

Normalized Polar Zernike Coefficients (µ)   High Order Aberrations Graph

	Value	Name	0.0	0.17109	Axis
Z_{20}	-1.02780	Defocus			
Z_{22}	0.36448 @ 170°	Astigmatism			
Z_{31}	0.12370 @ 220°	Coma			
Z_{33}	0.17109 @ 98°	Trefoil			
Z_{40}	0.06222	Sph. Aberration			
Z_{42}	0.06889 @ 4°				
Z_{44}	0.03261 @ 22°				
Z_{51}	0.02239 @ 343°				
Z_{53}	0.03482 @ 27°				
Z_{55}	0.07900 @ 66°				
Z_{60}	-0.00214				
Z_{62}	0.00546 @ 24°				
Z_{64}	0.03816 @ 5°				
Z_{66}	0.01533 @ 40°				

ILMO

3 SECTION

Right Eye Postoperative Aberrations Map

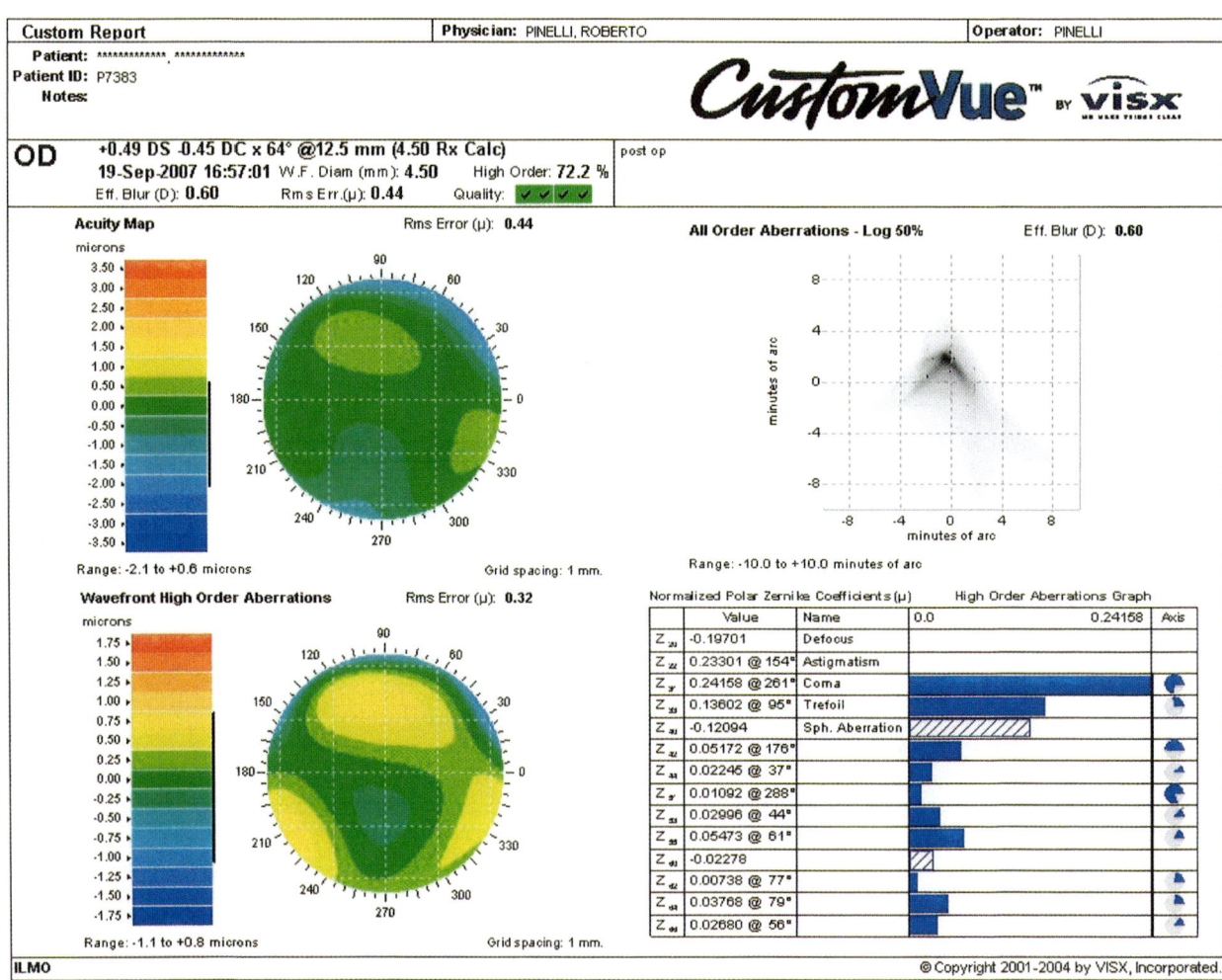

Left Eye Preoperative Aberrations Map

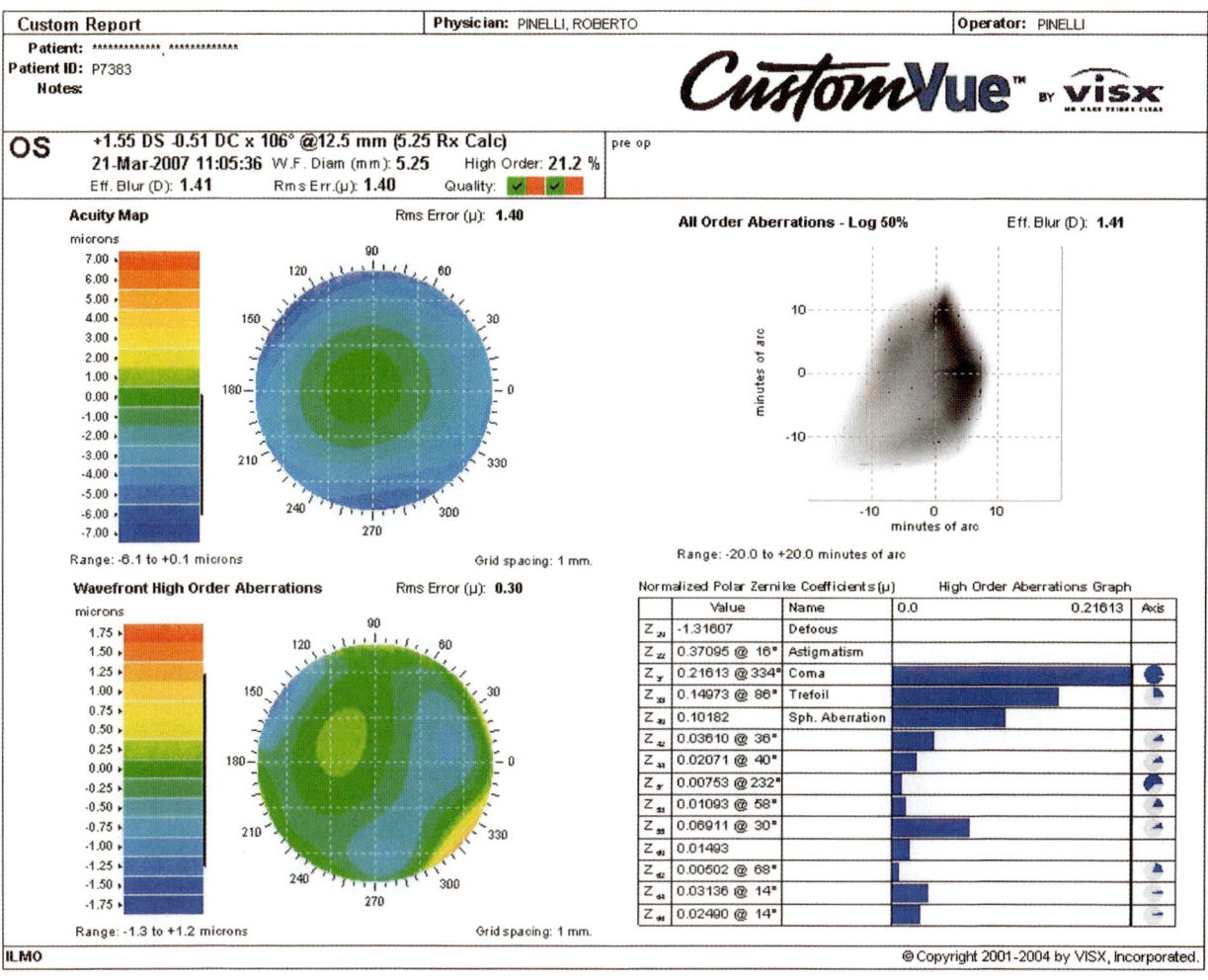

| | Custom Report | Physician: PINELLI, ROBERTO | Operator: PINELLI |

Patient: ************ ************
Patient ID: P7383
Notes:

CustomVue™ BY **VISX**

OS +1.55 DS -0.51 DC x 106° @12.5 mm (5.25 Rx Calc) pre op
21-Mar-2007 11:05:36 W.F. Diam (mm): **5.25** High Order: **21.2 %**
Eff. Blur (D): **1.41** Rms Err.(µ): **1.40** Quality: ✔ ✔

Acuity Map Rms Error (µ): **1.40**

microns
7.00
6.00
5.00
4.00
3.00
2.00
1.00
0.00
-1.00
-2.00
-3.00
-4.00
-5.00
-6.00
-7.00

Range: -6.1 to +0.1 microns   Grid spacing: 1 mm.

Wavefront High Order Aberrations Rms Error (µ): **0.30**

microns
1.75
1.50
1.25
1.00
0.75
0.50
0.25
0.00
-0.25
-0.50
-0.75
-1.00
-1.25
-1.50
-1.75

Range: -1.3 to +1.2 microns   Grid spacing: 1 mm.

All Order Aberrations - Log 50% Eff. Blur (D): **1.41**

Range: -20.0 to +20.0 minutes of arc

Normalized Polar Zernike Coefficients (µ) **High Order Aberrations Graph**

	Value	Name	0.0	0.21613	Axis
Z_{20}	-1.31607	Defocus			
Z_{22}	0.37095 @ 16°	Astigmatism			
Z_{31}	0.21613 @ 334°	Coma			
Z_{33}	0.14973 @ 86°	Trefoil			
Z_{40}	0.10182	Sph. Aberration			
Z_{42}	0.03610 @ 36°				
Z_{44}	0.02071 @ 40°				
Z_{51}	0.00753 @ 232°				
Z_{53}	0.01093 @ 58°				
Z_{55}	0.06911 @ 30°				
Z_{60}	0.01493				
Z_{62}	0.00502 @ 68°				
Z_{64}	0.03136 @ 14°				
Z_{66}	0.02490 @ 14°				

ILMO

Left Eye Postoperative Aberrations Map

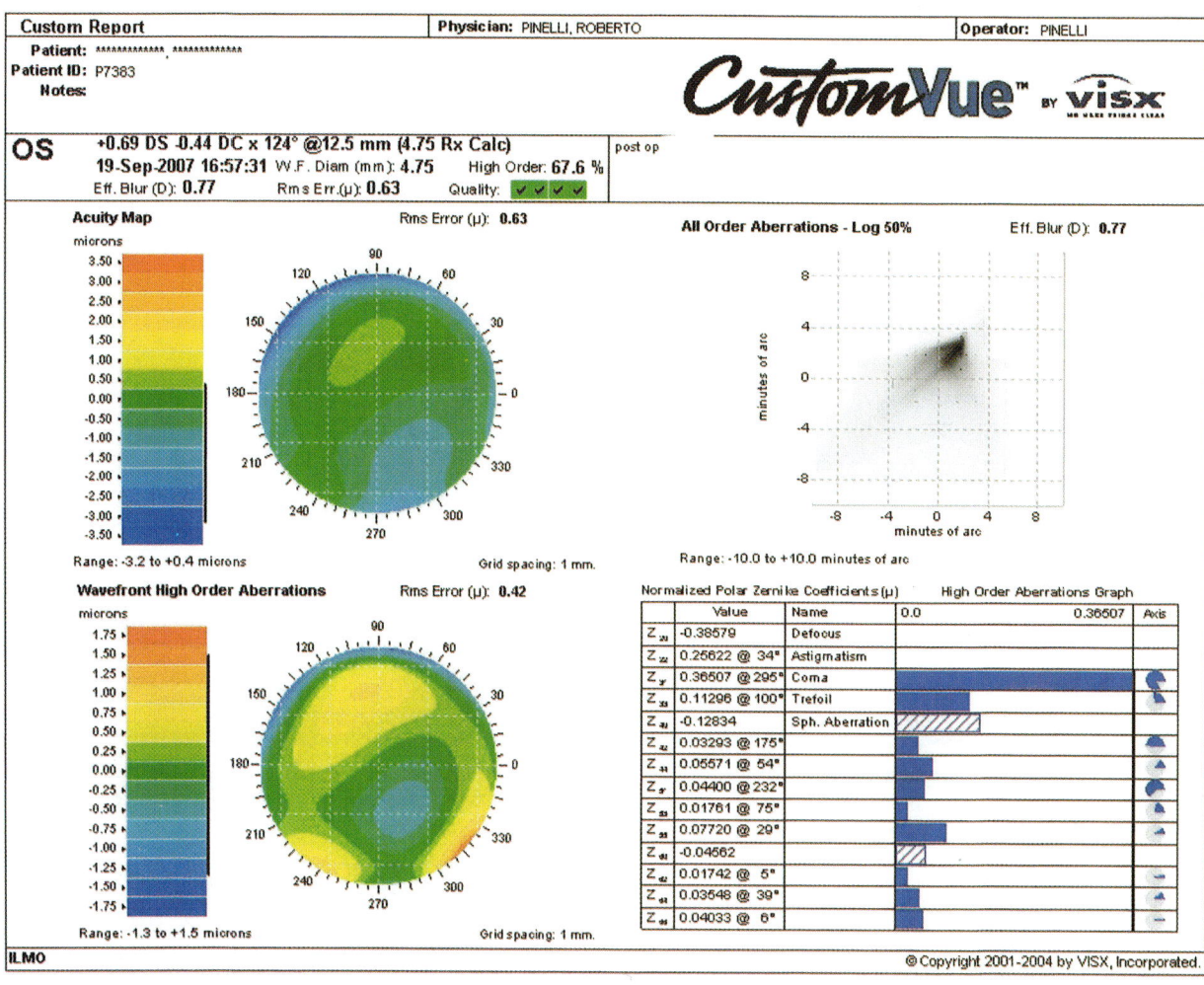

Custom Report	Physician: PINELLI, ROBERTO	Operator: PINELLI

Patient: ********** **********
Patient ID: P7383
Notes:

CustomVue™ BY **visx**

OS +0.69 DS -0.44 DC x 124° @12.5 mm (4.75 Rx Calc)   post op
19-Sep-2007 16:57:31 W.F. Diam (mm): 4.75   High Order: 67.6 %
Eff. Blur (D): 0.77   Rms Err.(µ): 0.63   Quality: ✔ ✔ ✔

Acuity Map   Rms Error (µ): 0.63

microns
3.50
3.00
2.50
2.00
1.50
1.00
0.50
0.00
-0.50
-1.00
-1.50
-2.00
-2.50
-3.00
-3.50

Range: -3.2 to +0.4 microns   Grid spacing: 1 mm.

All Order Aberrations - Log 50%   Eff. Blur (D): 0.77

Range: -10.0 to +10.0 minutes of arc

Wavefront High Order Aberrations   Rms Error (µ): 0.42

microns
1.75
1.50
1.25
1.00
0.75
0.50
0.25
0.00
-0.25
-0.50
-0.75
-1.00
-1.25
-1.50
-1.75

Range: -1.3 to +1.5 microns   Grid spacing: 1 mm.

Normalized Polar Zernike Coefficients (µ)   High Order Aberrations Graph

	Value	Name	0.0	0.36507	Axis
Z_{20}	-0.38579	Defocus			
Z_{22}	0.25622 @ 34°	Astigmatism			
$Z_{3'}$	0.36507 @ 295°	Coma			
Z_{33}	0.11296 @ 100°	Trefoil			
Z_{40}	-0.12834	Sph. Aberration			
Z_{42}	0.03293 @ 175°				
Z_{44}	0.05571 @ 54°				
$Z_{3'}$	0.04400 @ 232°				
Z_{33}	0.01761 @ 75°				
Z_{33}	0.07720 @ 29°				
Z_{60}	-0.04562				
Z_{62}	0.01742 @ 5°				
Z_{64}	0.03548 @ 39°				
Z_{66}	0.04033 @ 6°				

ILMO

CASE 5: Male, 56 years old

Preoperative UCVA for Far

RE: 20/50 nat
LE: 20/50 nat

Preoperative UCVA for Near

RE: J7 nat
LE: J7 nat

Preoperative BCVA for Far

RE: 20/20 sph. + 0.50 cyl + 0.75 ax 90°
LE: 20/20 sph. + 0.25 cyl + 0.75 ax 85°

Preoperative BCVA for Near

J1 add. +1.50 OU

Postoperative UCVA for Far (12 Months)

RE: 20/20
LE: 20/20

Autorefractometry Postoperative

RE: sph −0.75 cyl −0.25 ax 50°
LE: sph −0.50 cyl −0.50 ax 50°

Postoperative UCVA for Near

J1 OU.

SECTION 3

Right Eye Preoperative Aberrations Map

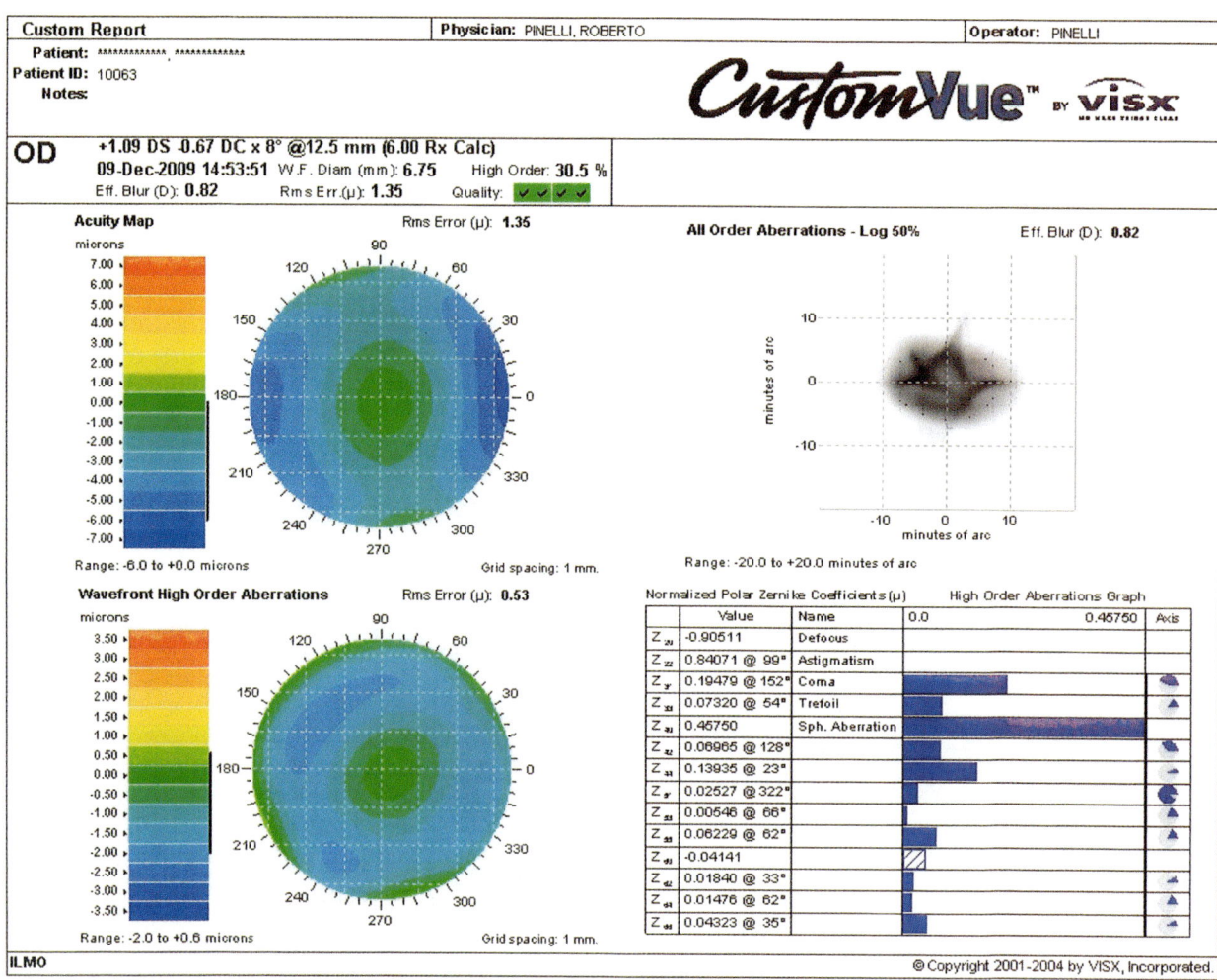

Custom Report | **Physician:** PINELLI, ROBERTO | **Operator:** PINELLI

Patient: ▮▮▮▮▮▮▮▮▮▮▮▮ ▮▮▮▮▮▮▮▮▮▮▮▮▮▮
Patient ID: 10063
Notes:

CustomVue ™ BY **visx** WE MAKE THINGS CLEAR

OD +1.09 DS -0.67 DC x 8° @12.5 mm (6.00 Rx Calc)
09-Dec-2009 14:53:51 W.F. Diam (mm): 6.75   High Order: 30.5 %
Eff. Blur (D): 0.82   Rms Err (μ): 1.35   Quality: ✓ ✓ ✓ ✓

Acuity Map   Rms Error (μ): 1.35

microns
7.00
6.00
5.00
4.00
3.00
2.00
1.00
0.00
-1.00
-2.00
-3.00
-4.00
-5.00
-6.00
-7.00

Range: -6.0 to +0.0 microns   Grid spacing: 1 mm.

All Order Aberrations - Log 50%   Eff. Blur (D): 0.82

Range: -20.0 to +20.0 minutes of arc

Wavefront High Order Aberrations   Rms Error (μ): 0.53

microns
3.50
3.00
2.50
2.00
1.50
1.00
0.50
0.00
-0.50
-1.00
-1.50
-2.00
-2.50
-3.00
-3.50

Range: -2.0 to +0.6 microns   Grid spacing: 1 mm.

Normalized Polar Zernike Coefficients (μ)   High Order Aberrations Graph

	Value	Name	0.0	0.45750	Axis
Z₂₀	-0.90511	Defocus			
Z₂₂	0.84071 @ 99°	Astigmatism			
Z₃₁	0.19479 @ 152°	Coma			
Z₃₃	0.07320 @ 54°	Trefoil			
Z₄₀	0.45750	Sph. Aberration			
Z₄₂	0.06965 @ 128°				
Z₄₄	0.13935 @ 23°				
Z₅₁	0.02527 @ 322°				
Z₅₃	0.00546 @ 66°				
Z₅₅	0.06229 @ 62°				
Z₆₀	-0.04141				
Z₆₂	0.01840 @ 33°				
Z₆₄	0.01476 @ 62°				
Z₆₆	0.04323 @ 35°				

ILMO

© Copyright 2001-2004 by VISX, Incorporated.

Right Eye Postoperative Aberrations Map

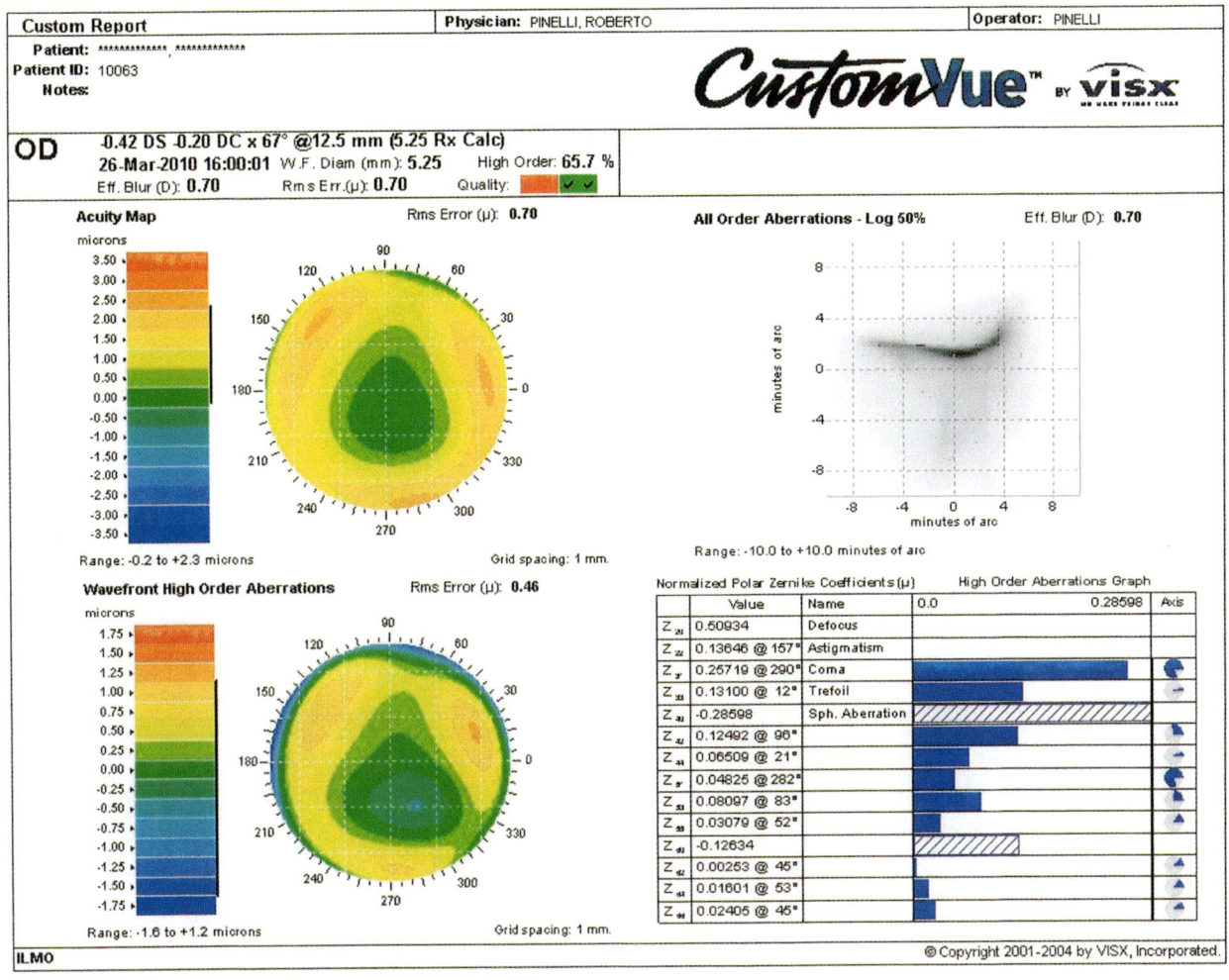

Left Eye Preoperative Aberrations Map

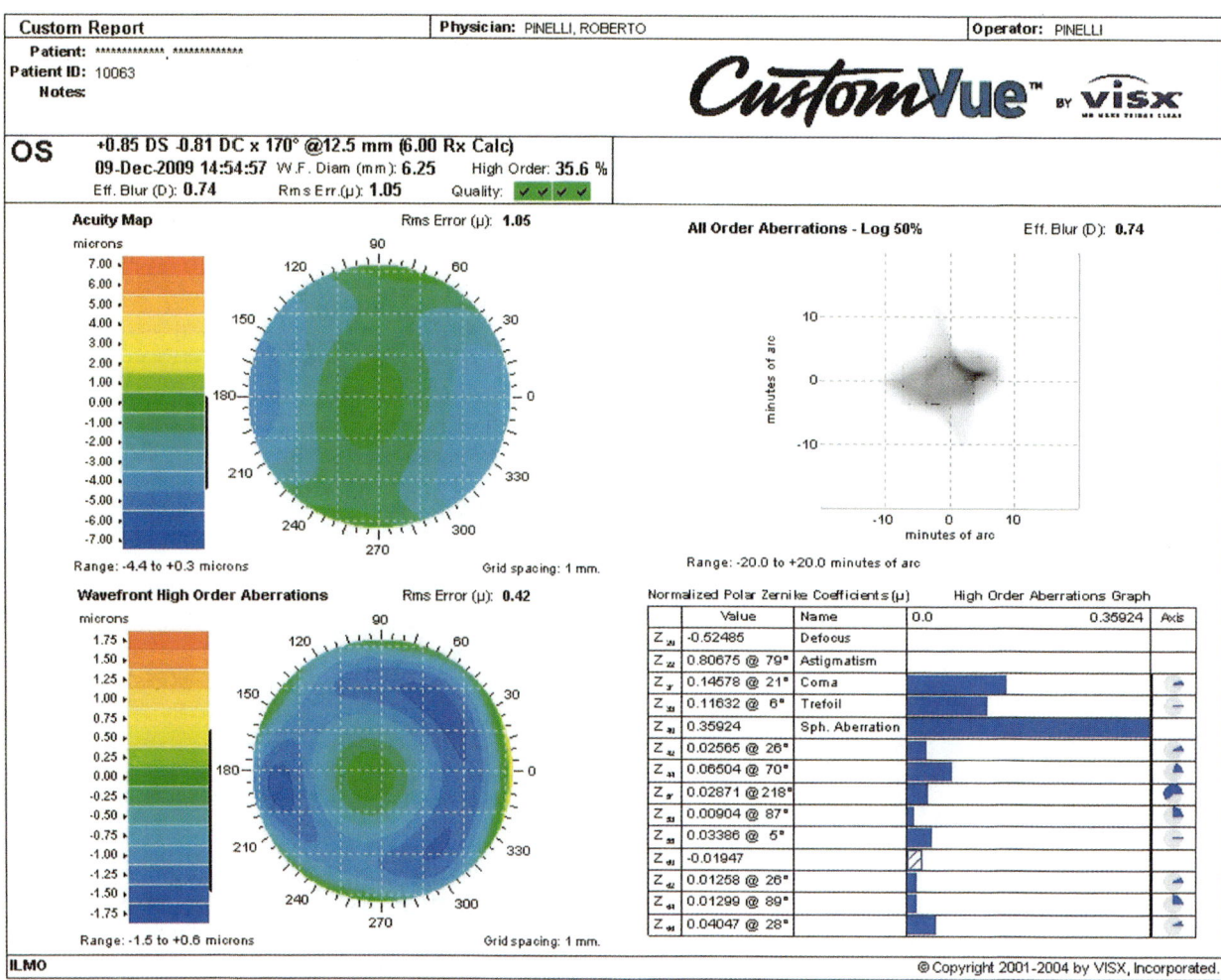

Left Eye Postoperative Aberrations Map

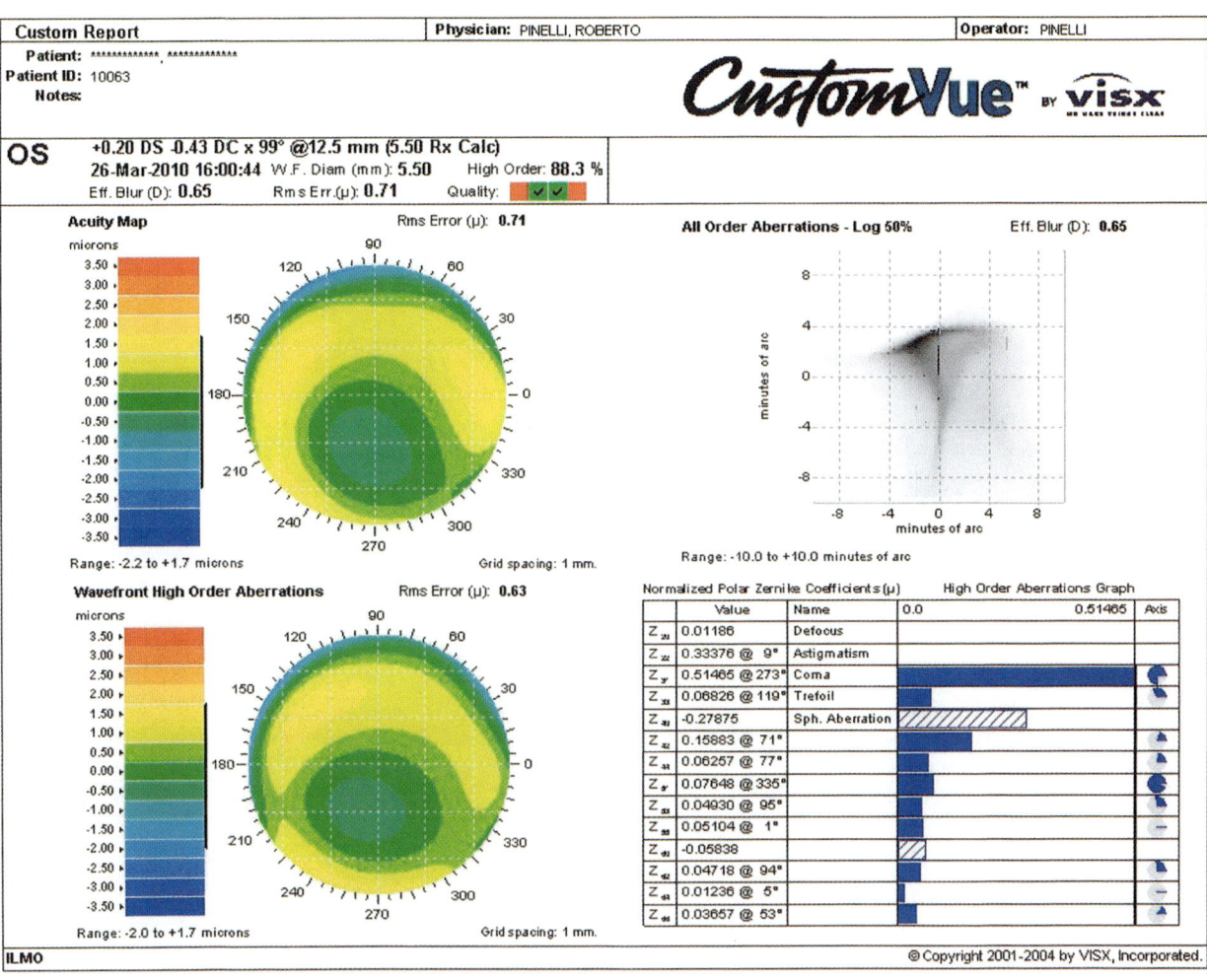

| | **Custom Report** | **Physician:** PINELLI, ROBERTO | **Operator:** PINELLI |

Patient: ************ ************
Patient ID: 10063
Notes:

CustomVue™ BY **visx** WE MAKE THINGS CLEAR

OS +0.20 DS -0.43 DC x 99° @12.5 mm (5.50 Rx Calc)
26-Mar-2010 16:00:44 W.F. Diam (mm): **5.50**   High Order: **88.3 %**
Eff. Blur (D): **0.65**   Rms Err.(µ): **0.71**   Quality: ✔ ✔

Acuity Map   Rms Error (µ): **0.71**

microns
3.50
3.00
2.50
2.00
1.50
1.00
0.50
0.00
-0.50
-1.00
-1.50
-2.00
-2.50
-3.00
-3.50

Range: -2.2 to +1.7 microns   Grid spacing: 1 mm.

All Order Aberrations - Log 50%   Eff. Blur (D): **0.65**

Range: -10.0 to +10.0 minutes of arc

Wavefront High Order Aberrations   Rms Error (µ): **0.63**

microns
3.50
3.00
2.50
2.00
1.50
1.00
0.50
0.00
-0.50
-1.00
-1.50
-2.00
-2.50
-3.00
-3.50

Range: -2.0 to +1.7 microns   Grid spacing: 1 mm.

Normalized Polar Zernike Coefficients (µ)   High Order Aberrations Graph

	Value	Name	0.0	0.51465	Axis
Z_{20}	0.01186	Defocus			
Z_{22}	0.33376 @ 9°	Astigmatism			
Z_{3f}	0.51465 @ 273°	Coma			
Z_{33}	0.06826 @ 119°	Trefoil			
Z_{40}	-0.27875	Sph. Aberration			
Z_{42}	0.15883 @ 71°				
Z_{44}	0.06257 @ 77°				
Z_{5f}	0.07648 @ 335°				
Z_{53}	0.04930 @ 95°				
Z_{55}	0.05104 @ 1°				
Z_{40}	-0.05838				
Z_{42}	0.04718 @ 94°				
Z_{44}	0.01236 @ 5°				
Z_{46}	0.03657 @ 53°				

ILMO   © Copyright 2001-2004 by VISX, Incorporated.

SECTION 4

Atlas

CHAPTER 12

Roberto Pinelli

Wavefront Basic Images

WHY THIS SIMPLE AND EMBLEMATIC ATLAS?

Lots of images are everyday running on our screens and diagnostic machines but some "clear" and "pure" images of aberrations, uncontaminated, will be more useful compared to a classic list. See the peculiarities of those "primordial" images. See also the power of those pure designs and think with your own knowledge and mind to the symbolic message of those. And do not forget, when, if we use them, we always create a compromise. This small and primordial Atlas is an invitation/suggestion/intimidation to think that we are playing with great concepts.

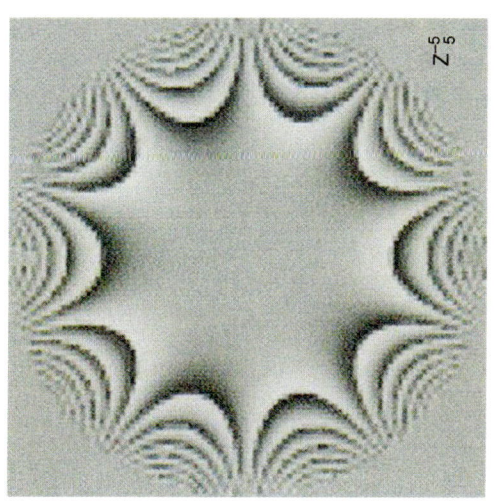

Pentafoil

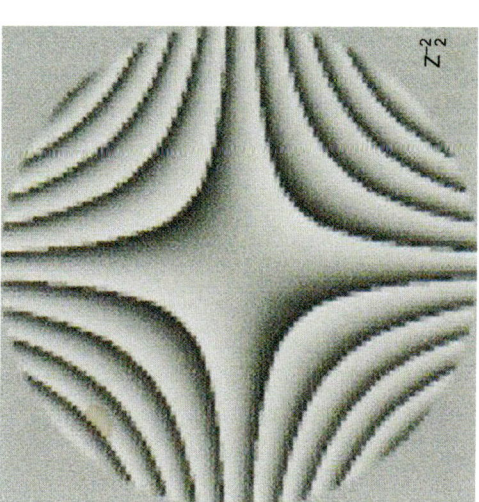

Astigmatism

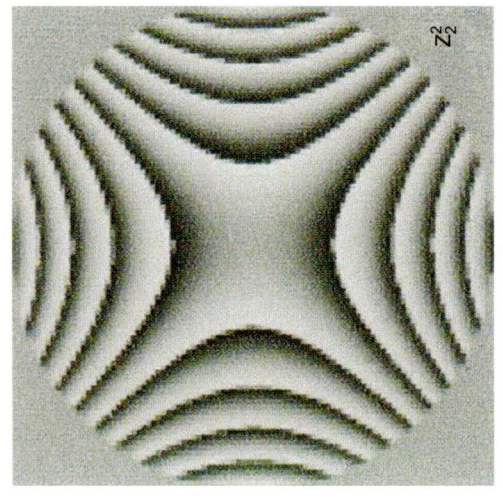

Astigmatism

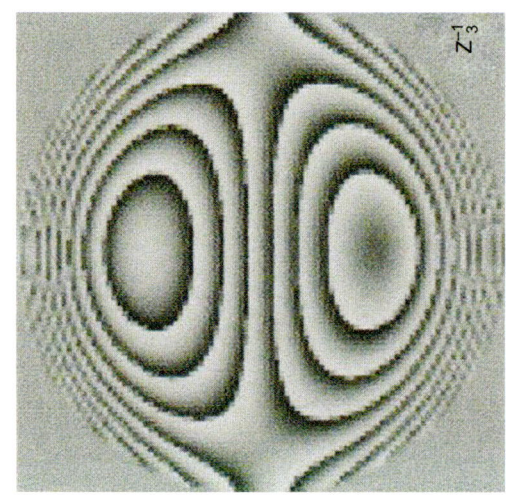

Coma

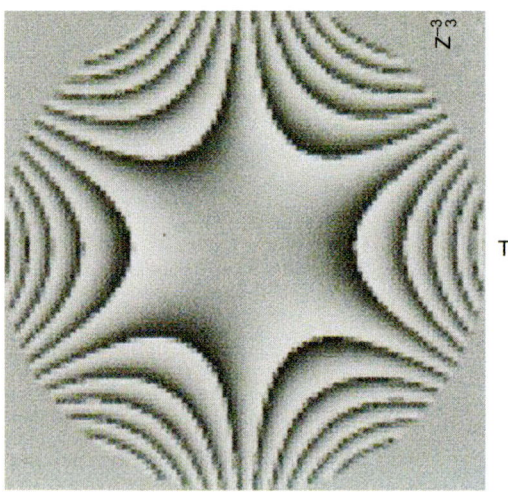

Trefoil

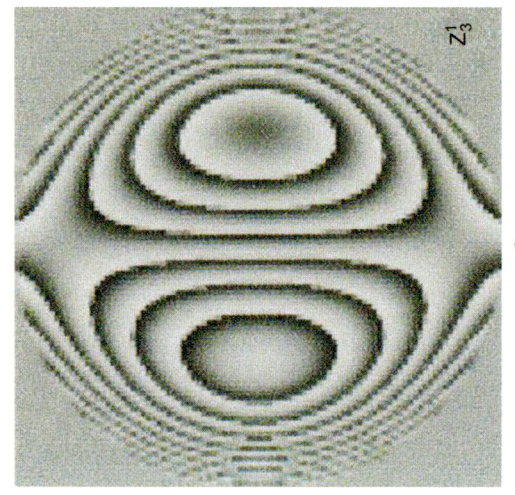

Coma

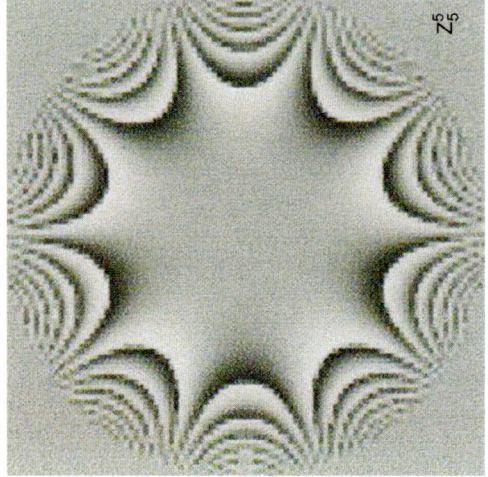

Pentafoil

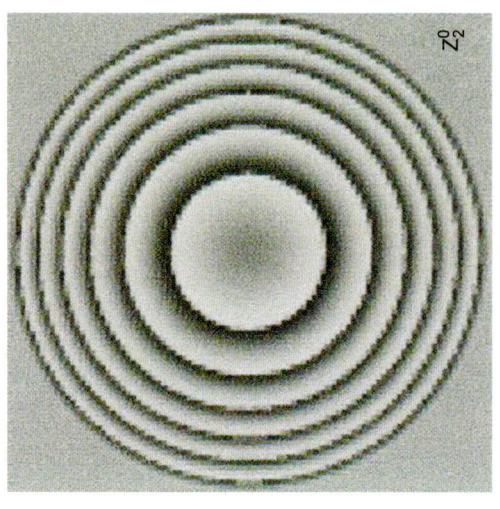

Defocus

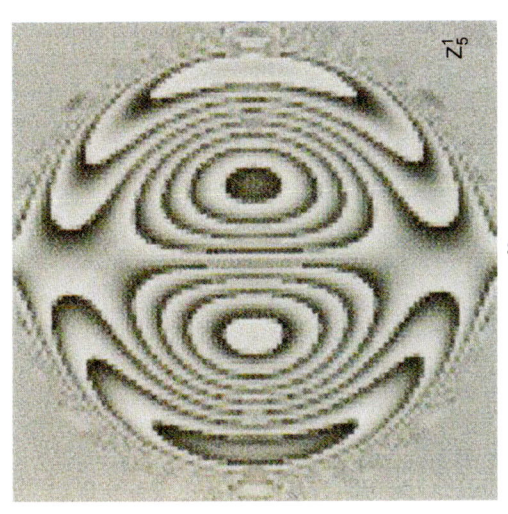

Secondary
coma

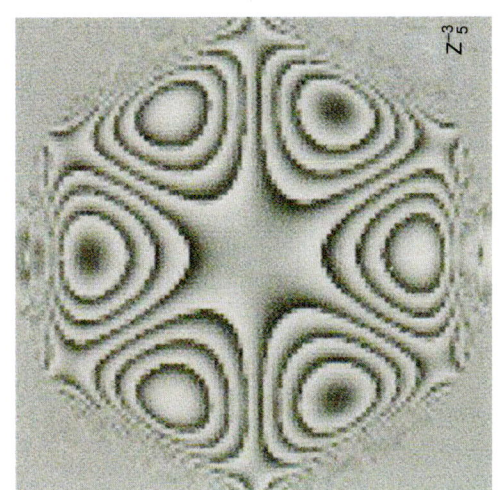

Secondary
trefoil

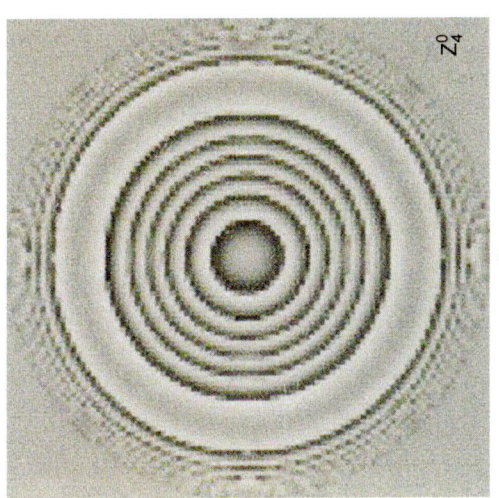

Spherical

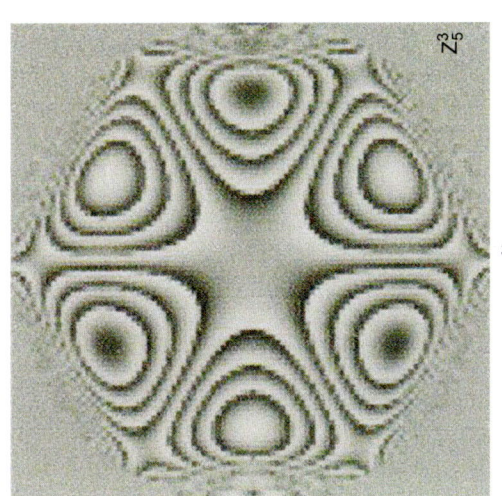

Secondary
trefoil

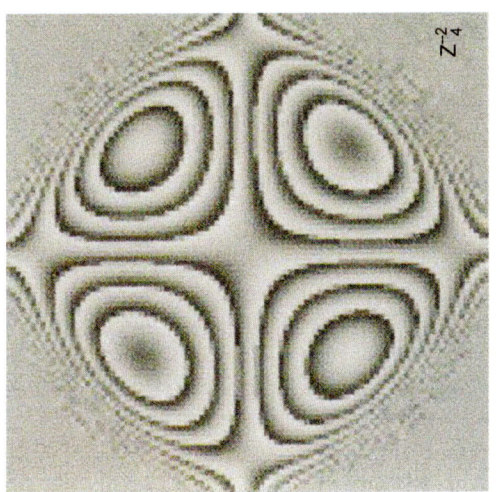

Secondary
astigmatism

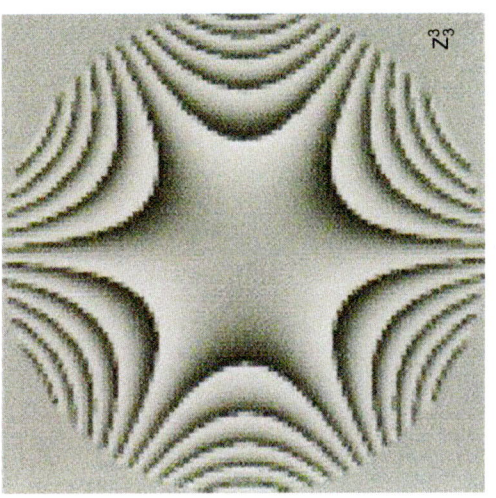

Trefoil

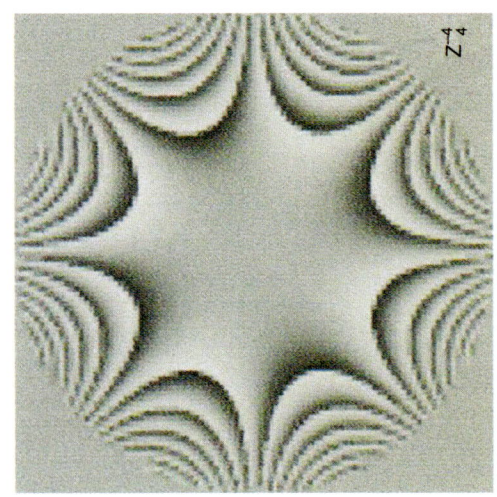

Z_4^{-4}

Quadrafoil

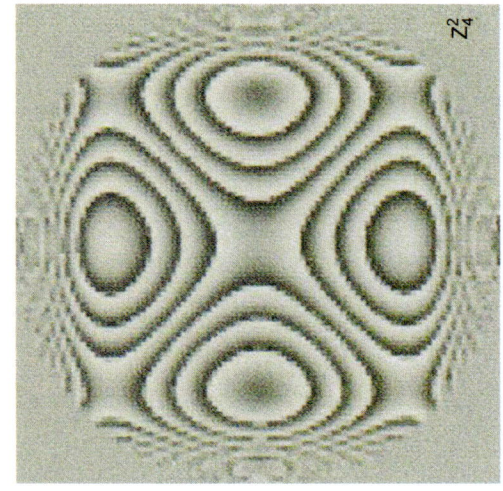

Z_4^2

Secondary astigmatism

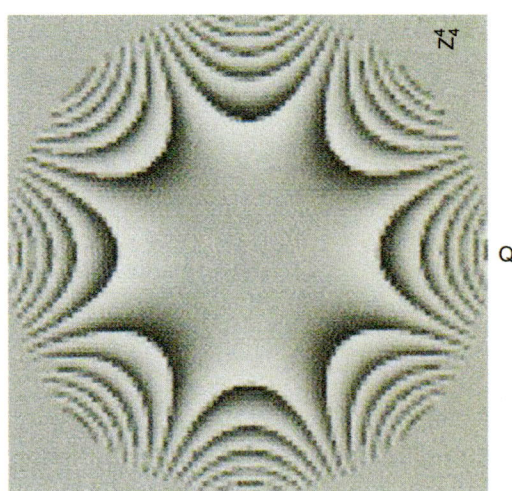

Z_4^4

Quadrafoil

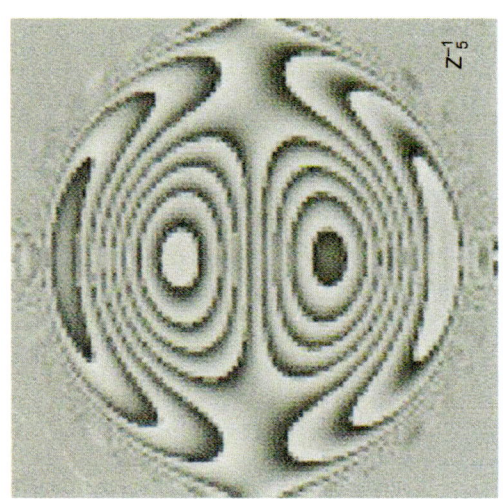

Z_5^{-1}

Secondary coma

Index

Page numbers followed by *f* refer to figure